DeeDee Jameson is Assistant Professor of Early Childhood and Human Development in the School of Home Economics at the University of Vermont. She is presently involved in study which will enable her to design a Life Center providing a community for those interested in self-help and shared responsibility for children. She lives in Jericho, Vermont.

Roberta Schwalb is a registered nurse and certified nurse midwife. She is currently Associate Professor of professional nursing at the University of Vermont and is an experienced teacher and practitioner of Obstetrical and Gynecological Nursing. She lives in Williston, Vermont.

EVERY WOMAN'S GUIDE TO HYSTERECTOMY
Taking Charge of Your Own Body

DEEDEE JAMESON
ROBERTA SCHWALB, R.N., C.N.M.

A SPECTRUM BOOK

PRENTICE-HALL, INC., Englewood Cliffs, N.J. 07632

Library of Congress Cataloging in Publication Data

JAMESON, DEEDEE.
    Every woman's guide to hysterectomy.

    (A Spectrum Book)
    Bibliography: p.
    1. Hysterectomy. I. Schwalb, Roberta, joint
author. II. Title. [DNLM: 1. Hysterectomy—
Popular works. WP468 J31e]
RG391.J35   618.1 ′453   77-14339
ISBN 0-13-292821-3
ISBN 0-13-292813-2 pbk.

© 1978 by Prentice-Hall, Inc., Englewood Cliffs, N.J. 07632

A SPECTRUM BOOK

Printed in the United States of America

10 9 8 7 6 5 4 3 2 1

PRENTICE-HALL INTERNATIONAL, INC., *London*
PRENTICE-HALL OF AUSTRALIA PTY., LIMITED, *Sydney*
PRENTICE-HALL OF CANADA, LTD., *Toronto*
PRENTICE-HALL OF INDIA PRIVATE, LIMITED, *New Delhi*
PRENTICE-HALL OF JAPAN, INC., *Tokyo*
PRENTICE-HALL OF SOUTHEAST ASIA PTE., LTD., *Singapore*
WHITEHALL BOOKS, LIMITED, *Wellington, New Zealand*

*This book is dedicated to the
"new beginnings" which are possible
for each of us.*

Contents

Foreword

Every Woman's Guide to Hysterectomy: Taking Charge of Your Own Body is a thought provoking, timely and helpful book for women contemplating this operation and those who care for these women. Moreover, it has a message for all women who expect or are expected to take more responsibility for themselves with reference to their own well-being.

Hysterectomy is controversial in large part because of the responsibility women want and are taking for their own bodies and health care. Little more than a decade ago, the indications [medical reasons] for having this operation were fairly cut and dried. Any modification of indication during the previous half-century was primarily due to increasing the safety factor, so that as time went on, hysterectomy could be performed when it was considered advisable, rather than only as a life-saving procedure. However, until ten years ago, there were still more or less absolute indications as defined by gynecologic practice and accepted by most patients. There was no total agreement upon indication, but criticism was primarily focused on the fact that physicians did not adhere to the traditional guidelines.

During the last decade a virtual revolution has taken place. Indications have been considerably modified because women have made it clear that they want something to say about anything as personal as removal of a uterus. In addition, some newly accepted indications such as sterilization have made it mandatory that the patient be a responsible partner in deciding upon the procedure. In this situation the clinician can best assist the patient in making what seems to be a valid and good decision based upon what the patient describes in her medical history. Since many women and their physicians hold diverse opinions about the increasing partnership of women, it is no wonder that the subject of hysterectomy is involved in turmoil. The book provides a calm, instructive approach which should be of help to patients in their decision-making and to physicians in their considerations.

One of the more valuable parts of this book is DeeDee Jameson's *Journal.* I found this section of great significance to me as a physician because she points out vividly how important an operation is to the patient and her family. This may be forgotten by physicians, nurses and other hospital personnel. It is easy for professionals who are involved in operations on a daily basis to forget exactly how patients and families feel.

The fact that an operation is so important to those closely involved makes them very vulnerable. To me, it is a given fact that vulnerability should be protected, and that the patient receive compassion and understanding. The journal points out the real anguish of a patient approaching an operation. At one point DeeDee said she "just hoped I would be alive in a week," and "they did not understand how frightened I was." Physicians need to be reminded of patients' concerns and act accordingly. Perhaps what Oliver Wendell Holmes said about mothers should be applied generally to all patients:

> The woman about to become a mother, or with her new-born infant upon her bosom, should be the object of trembling care and sympathy wherever she bears her tender burden or stretches her aching limbs—God forbid that any member of the profession to which she trust her life, doubly precious at that eventful period, should hazard it negligently, unadvisedly or selfishly.

Other parts of the book should be particularly helpful to patients who are involved with a decision regarding hysterectomy. Bobbie Schwalb outlined in clear fashion some of the steps in deciding about hysterectomy: defining the problem, analyzing information, considering alternatives, and exploring alternatives with others. Idealistically, I believe that the physician should help the patient with the first three and also suggest that she discuss the alternatives with her family and close associates. Certainly no step should be omitted but a problem may arise because, in my experience, some patients want to explore their own condition in greater depth than others. Everyone should have the right to know as much as they want but I do not believe information should be forced upon the patient any more than it should be withheld.

This question of inadequate information is something that needs more thought. At one point, DeeDee said that she didn't know enough to ask the proper questions and was reluctant to express the feeling that she did not feel informed. It is unfortunate that we are often unable to express feelings, because it has been my observation that the expression of feelings can overcome lack of knowledge in finding the proper solution. It would be helpful to patients if they tried to express their feelings more and if physicians would actively encourage patients to express feelings. DeeDee's experience with the medical student who had compassion and sympathy rather than great knowledge was illuminating.

Finally, some parts of the book would seem to be valuable for both patients and physicians. I was moved by Bobbie Schwalb's discussion of hospital environment as one in which there is a loss of freedom, loss of control and a loss of identity. Virtually everyone who has ever been a patient can identify with these feelings. Having recently been a hospital patient, I know that I can. The fact that I was a physician and a patient in my own hospital made less difference than one would suppose. Certainly, things can be done to make patients more comfortable in an emotional way through a concerted joint effort among patients, physicians, and hospital administration. A particularly fine quality of this book is that it spells out problems and feelings in a very direct and non-hostile way.

This is a book that can make a difference! I hope all of us utilize it to do so.

R. CLAY BURCHELL, M.D.
Dept. of Obstetrics and Gynecology
Hartford Hospital
Hartford, Connecticut

Preface

This book is our way of sharing some very important ideas with you. It could be called a very private story, and it is. But there is a dimension of commonality which leads us to believe that this is your story, too.

Our point of focus is hysterectomy. This is significant because *it is the second most frequently performed surgery in our country* (tonsilectomy is first). Almost three-quarters of a million women undergo this surgery each year. Twelve thousand of them will die. Over half of the women in our country who are over forty will be advised to have their wombs removed. Of the women who undergo this surgery, over half will lose their ovaries and fallopian tubes.[1]

---

[1] *National Health Survey,* "Surgical Operations in Short-Stay Hospitals" (Rockville, Md.: U.S. DHEW Publ. No. (HRA) 76-1775, U.S. 1973) Series 13, No. 14, May 1976, p. 9.

But this book is about more than the surgery itself. In addition to supplying accurate information about hysterectomy, we suggest that *you* are the person who has the right and obligation to assume responsibility for the care of your body. There are specific suggestions for action and resources for you to turn to—there can be more. But you must inform yourself and use some initiative in seeking out support for yourself.

Each of you who reads this book will have a different motivation for reading it; you will bring different questions with you; you each have a special and unique background. Perhaps you are curious and concerned because your wife or mother or friend has been advised to undergo hysterectomy. Maybe you are a student in health care or human development and you would like to develop a more sensitive understanding of the whole issue of female surgery. You might be a person interested in the improvement of health care delivery in the area of administration, politics or education, or in all of these.

You may be a woman who has some initial feelings that this book was meant for you. You won't all be the same age. Some of you are facing this awareness at a very young age. In terms of child-bearing and aging this growing awareness can be a terribly painful process.

Some of you are feeling very, very afraid because your situation is not one which allows you any choice. You are in need of a great deal of support—now, and in the time to come.

And what about those of you who aren't used to using a lot of initiative to seek out the help you need? Maybe the system, in one way or another, has defeated you so many times that you have long since given up.

This book cannot provide all the answers for everyone. We have tried to provide some answers and some ways to gain insight and understanding. We think that the best thing we have done is to open up communication, to provide some specific ideas for action, and to help you begin to identify resources.

For those of you who are very private people, use this book for the kinds of information and support you need. For those of you who are able to reach out to others, try contactiong your local Woman's Health Center and find other people who might like to develop an "interest and support" group.

For those of you who have almost given up, *please don't give up*. Turn to people. They are there, wherever you live. Try your Woman's Health Center. If there isn't one in your area, look to such local groups as family health centers, Visiting Nurses Association, day care centers, churches—especially those churches that have taken a positive stand on human issues and get involved in action.

You see, we all start out in life with this wonderful gift—a human body. Touching it, feeling it, knowing it—all these experiences provide us with our first awareness of ourselves. Our bodies truly belong to us—no one else. They are our initial source of identity, our source of strength and enjoyment, our very personal responsibility.

Once you accept and understand this idea and start to live it in your daily life, you will see that it begins to spread out into a lot of ways you feel about yourself. This book focuses on hysterectomy. It treats the many issues which are involved. But the premise is that once *you* take responsibility for yourself and begin to do something about your own decisions and development, you are on your way to something very special: a new beginning.

Acknowledgments

The writing of this book has been an exciting cooperative effort. Together the authors collected the many "Resources" which close the book. Together they wrote "You! A Member of Your Health Team" and "Today Is the First Day. . . ."

Bobbie Schwalb authored "Participating in the Decision" and "Your Hospital Stay: Admission to Discharge." The Preface, the "Journal," "Kiss Cinderella Goodbye," and "Today" were written by DeeDee Jameson.

For reading and editing sections of the manuscript we express our appreciation to Faith Emerson, Julie Jameson, Linda Richard, Danielle Lapointe, and John Eckerson. The skill and tireless efforts of Shirley Tetreault and Lucille Sargent made it possible to meet many of our deadlines with the manuscript. We thank Janet Patterson and Lydia Mayer for their help in the early planning stages of this book. And a very special thanks goes to Armin Grams and Larry Shelton, who had every faith that this book would be written and published. With the support of these good people, the writing of this book was a shared adventure.

DEEDEE JAMESON
BOBBIE SCHWALB
Burlington, Vermont

JOURNAL

We know that you will identify with many of the thoughts and feelings which are shared in this description of one woman's experience.

AWARENESS

October, 1972

Nowhere on earth is it more beautiful at this time of year than in my Vermont. The afternoon sun was warm today—but not like summer. Leaves swirled everywhere about my feet, reminding me that God's gift of color here and in the hills would soon fade, leaving many trees ready to spend the winter at rest.

More than a quarter century has passed since I came here to live—spanning my life from young womanhood into middle age.

I walked toward the administration building on the campus where I teach. Recently elected to a position of leadership, I had been asked to attend a meeting which would help me learn more about how a university is operated.

The meeting opened a whole new world for me. I made a mental note that I was the only woman present. Other business made it necessary for me to excuse myself before the meeting was over. As I stood up to leave the room, I felt a sudden warm gush and I realized that it had happened again. I had passed a blood clot.

Fortunately, the bathroom was right down the hall. I was wearing a sanitary napkin although my monthly period had just ended. For a few months now I've had some problems—but nothing like this. I was bleeding heavily.

I bought two napkins from the vending machine and tried to clean myself up. There was a huge stain on my skirt. The blood seemed to be running out of me. I fet very upset and I was scared. Because showers had been forecast, I had my slicker with me. I put it on, made my way to the parking lot, and drove to my doctor's office a block or two away.

No one at the doctor's office was concerned when I explained what was happening and expressed my fears. Although the staff was courteous and efficient, I felt that they did not understand how frightened I was. I was sure I was hemorrhaging. The doctor was not there, and that added to my feelings of insecurity.

One of the nurses helped me to clean myself up and then sent me to the appointment desk to arrange to see the doctor in a week. I just hoped that I would be alive in a week. It felt as though I would bleed to death before I got home.

Tonight I feel unsure and annoyed. Why did this have to happen to me? Everything had been going so well until this mess started two or three months ago.

The Interim Week

I will be going to the doctor's tomorrow. This feels like it has been the longest week in my life. The bleeding finally stopped and I feel like cancelling the appointment. I'd like to pretend that the whole thing was a figment of my imagination. That's my emotional self. My rational self knows that there is a problem and that I'd better tend to it.

As this past week crept along—day by terrible day—I thought back through the years, remembering some of the experiences of my life as a female. I remembered when I first learned about "the curse." I was about twelve years old. Daddy was out of town, and it was my turn to sleep in his bed and be Mother's roommate. My younger sister and I considered this experience a real treat! Mother and I always chatted awhile in the darkened room before going to sleep. This night, she was strangely quiet. I thought her voice seemed different when she finally spoke.

"DeeDee, I have something to tell you. Do you remember when you were younger that I told you that when Daddy and I wanted a baby, we prayed to God and He answered our prayers and planted a seed in me and that seed grew into a baby and you were born?"

"Yes." I did remember that.

"Well, that wasn't quite the way it happened."

There was quite a long period of silence, and I was sure that something very mysterious was going on. I also wondered what really did happen. Finally, Mother started talking again.

"When you get a little older, your body will start to make a seed every month. But you won't have any babies until you grow up and get married. The seed will pass out of your body every month and there will be blood. That is called 'having your period.' It isn't anything for you to worry about. Just tell me when it happens, and I will show you how to take care of yourself."

Eventually I asked Mother how it was that the seed could grow into a baby when you got married. Her voice had that different sound again, and she said it was the husband that was able to make this happen. She told me to be very careful around boys because it was important not to have babies until you got married. I wasn't at all sure what being "careful" around boys meant. But I was certain that I should not push for more specific information.

6

Later I learned that because several girls at the high school had gotten pregnant, my parents had decided that this was the time for my lesson. My father believed that it was Mother's responsibility to warn my sister and me and keep us virgins. I have often wondered what his lesson to a son would have been like, if he had had a son.

In my musings this past week, I also recalled the day that the big moment arrived. The month was March—two months after I turned thirteen. I was practicing the piano and felt a cramping sensation. I went to the bathroom and discovered some blood on the toilet tissue.

I remember running downstairs, feeling very excited, and calling out, "I'm a woman. Mother! I'm a woman!"

There was a repairman working in the kitchen. Mother looked a little embarrassed. She took me upstairs and showed me how to use a sanitary pad and belt and how to take care of myself. She was careful to caution me that this was a private matter and was not to be discussed with others.

Throughout my adolescent years, my menstrual periods were erratic and almost always accompanied by severe cramps. It was made quite clear that this was a part of my life which should never be discussed with males. In spite of all this, I never really felt it was a curse. It was always a very reassuring time. It always seemed very normal to me. It became an important part of how I perceived myself as a female.

I am sure that this is at the bottom of some of the anxious feelings I am experiencing right now. Something is wrong and I know it. I am troubled because of this. I want to ignore it and hope it will go away. I don't want to face the likelihood that it won't.

As I sit here tonight, I cannot help but wonder if this is the beginning of menopause for me. I really don't want to think about it. But I am forty-four years old. I think back to something that happened two years ago.

I had gotten home from work, feeling strung-out and pressured. Being a single parent of five active kids can be a real challenge at times. Demands were being placed on me one after another this particular evening. I let things build up too long and finally blew my stack.

Once things settled down and I had control of myself again, we all sat down to talk things out and share our feelings. My oldest child—actually a young woman—said that they were studying some things in her senior class in high school that helped her to understand me.

"I really know how you feel right now, Mother," she said. "You are going through the menopause, and you are having problems with your hormone balance. You can't help it if you lose your temper."

I remember denying that unconditionally. With finality I claimed that I would never have that problem. I was to busy to "go through" menopause. It would simply have to wait.

Tonight I am not so sure. I cannot deny that routine, cyclic patterns are changing. But it is hard to move into another phase of my development. I'm not ready for that. . . .

The Appointment

You know how it is when you make an appointment to see a doctor because something is bothering you and then, when the time for the appointment arrives, that "something" goes away and you feel foolish taking up his time? That is how I felt today when I saw my doctor.

He came into the examination room, smiling and friendly. He is a reassuring person and I know that he is competent. I trust him. This is very important to me.

We began to discuss what was happening to me. He listened intently as I went over my history. After the birth of my first child, just about nineteen years ago, my monthly periods became regular and very predictable. They were spaced about thirty days apart. They lasted five or six days, with the flow heavy the first three days, then slowing down to almost nothing the last day or two. The severe cramps of my earlier years were nonexistent.

About three months ago, I began to experience some changes. I started to have unexpected bleeding in between my periods. The periods seemed to come out of cycle, sometimes in three weeks, sometimes in five. I really could not depend on a schedule any longer. What was even more upsetting was that I often passed small clots.

"I really feel silly being here today," I said. "That problem I had last week was the worse time I've had. But the bleeding stopped and I feel very good now."

"You shouldn't feel that way," he reassured me. "You are doing the right thing in being here."

After the examination, we continued our discussion. "What you are experiencing is not uncommon to women your age," he explained. "You know that there are fibroid tumors present in your uterus. There have been for some time. I suggest that you make an appointment to see me in six months. If you are still experiencing this heavy bleeding when you return, we can try a D & C before we consider a hysterectomy."

Terrible feelings engulfed me. A hysterectomy? Of all the worries and concerns I had, including menopause, a hysterectomy had never been one of them.

"A hysterectomy? You can't possibly be thinking of doing that to me! I'm a healthy woman. It isn't normal to remove the reproductive system of a healthy woman. Even my kids know about the hormone balance of women my age. I don't want to grow old suddenly—ahead of my time. . . ." I said none of this. I am not sure why. I think I felt the need to keep up a courageous front.

Instead of talking, I simply took all those feelings home with me and lived with them for the next few months.

A Long Winter

It is spring now in Vermont. The rain falls in a steady, gentle shower some days. At other times it comes in bursts. Always it serves a purpose by melting the snow in high places and filling our wells and springs.

I think that living in this very special place has helped me to get through the long winter this year. I live on a dirt road in an old farmhouse that was built over one hundred years ago. I look out my front windows onto two beautiful mountains. They were here long before I was born; they will be here long after I die. Knowing this helps me to keep my life in perspective. I am important because I am. But I recognize that I have only one small place in the scheme of things.

My physical condition has remained about the same. The unpredictable timing of my menstrual periods, the intermittent and heavy bleeding, and the fairly regular clotting have remained a part of my condition. I feel anxious about this.

During the winter, I have tried to concentrate on the positive. Having children was very important to me. And I had them—five of them in seven years, with two miscarriages in between. Sounds irresponsible to me now as I think about the population problems we have on this earth. But I am a responsible parent, and with the help of many good people in our community, the kids have grown to be healthy, bright, and caring human beings.

Still, I am experiencing anxieties about what

is happening to my body. I must either wear or take sanitary napkins with me most of the time now. It is difficult to plan on anything. I find that the active nature of my work often makes more demands than I can cope with. I tell myself that I'd like another six years. Maybe when I hit fifty, I'll be ready for this.

If it's menopause, I've decided that I'm not going to "go through it." My mother did that, and all I remember was twenty years of hell. Once, when my sister and I were adults and had homes of our own, she said that the years when we were children were the best years of her life.

Now that disturbs me. My mother will be seventy years old this summer. She spent less than twenty-five years of her life actively mothering us, too long at that. What about the other two-thirds of her life? Weren't those years worth something? I have to believe they were. I have to believe that there is a DeeDee after motherhood.

If it's hysterectomy—well, I'm less prepared to face that. It is so sudden and involves so many other fears. I keep reminding myself that we can try the D & C first. I've had two of those—after the miscarriages. I feel secure about that alternative. Maybe I'll have those six years yet!

MAKING A DECISION

May 18, 1973

I went for my regular checkup today. It was really a relief to have a routine appointment. The doctor said to call if there were any changes or if I felt concerned. But I have never felt comfortable doing that. Maybe it's just my personality, but I have always thought that doctors are such busy people that I shouldn't bother them unless I'm at death's door.

And, honestly, I wasn't sure what was cause for concern. Maybe my experience was nothing more than a routine progression for a middle-aged woman with fibroid tumors. I was sure that the next step was a D & C. Because I have unlimited faith—or false hope—I was sure this would correct my problem. I would be my good old earthy self again—all woman.

After announcing my arrival to the receptionist, I was asked to sit down and wait. I looked over the magazines that were arranged neatly on a rack. Most of them had to do with making homes beautiful or having and raising babies.

A nurse called my name and asked me to follow her. I clutched my magazine tightly. I don't know why, but I am always afraid that some nurse or receptionist is going to ask me where I think I'm going with that magazine. But I have learned to have something to read when the nurse leaves with the statement, ''The doctor will be with you in just a minute or so.''

After changing clothes, I used the bathroom, being sure to leave a urine sample in the flask which appears and disappears quite mysteriously, working its own wonders. You know that the system works because you are billed for it.

The nurse led me into an examination room, and I climbed onto the table. She took my blood pressure which I assume was normal. At least she didn't gasp. The famous prick came next, and a few spindles of blood were drawn off. Those little spindles always remind me of the perfume samples which are given away at conventions for the men to give to their "ladies." Anyway, the spindles of blood also disappeared mysteriously—to join the flask of urine, no doubt—never to be heard of again, except on the invoice.

Her part of the examination done, the nurse left with the message, "The doctor will be with you in just a minute or so." Out with the magazine!

Eventually my doctor came into the room. He was warm and friendly, as he always is, patient and willing to answer questions. But I don't think I knew enough to ask the necessary questions.

We went the route of routine information together, and in the process, I was able to share the knowledge that my situation had certainly not improved. The examination followed the discussion period. The examination is the biggest mystery of all.

I have always felt lucky that there are such nice posters on the ceiling. This morning I read them and tried to relax and forget, for a little while, that I didn't know what was happening to me. I knew that I would have to lie down and slide down, way down, to the end of the table. I am always terrified that I will fall off. Due to some kind of puritanical heritage, a sheet prevented me from being able to see what was happening to me. Luckily my doctor is the type who keeps up a kind of running commentary. But this commentary is nonspecific, and I only know what I can feel. Mostly this is some kind of cold, metal tool which is placed in my vagina and screwed open. It made me feel as though this were the moment to rinse, dry well, salt, and place the stuffing in loosely.

When the examination was over, my doctor cleaned me off and threw all of the paraphernalia, including his gloves, into the step-on garbage can. Once again I came back from the jaws of death and slid from the end of that table into an upright position. We began to talk.

As we discussed the fact that I was still experiencing heavy and unpredictable bleeding, it became obvious that we both felt something had to be done about this. I was attentive as he outlined the procedures in terms of the plans I would have to make. He mentioned that I would be in the hospital for about a week. I knew that a week's stay in the hospital was not necessary for a D & C.

"You aren't talking about a D & C?" I asked.

"No, that wouldn't really take care of your problem. I'm talking about a hysterectomy."

There was that word again. I felt just awful sitting there. I couldn't believe this was necessary. I am in good health and only forty-five years old.

"How much of a hysterectomy? Will I lose my ovaries, too?"

"Probably. We can wait to see how healthy they are when we are in surgery. With a younger woman, we try to save at least one ovary. But with a woman your age, we generally find that the ovaries need to come out. And we like to avoid having you go through surgery again, in a few years, to have them out later."

The room seemed so quiet. I tried desperately

to stall for time. All kinds of thoughts raced through my head. Maybe the clotting and unpredictable bleeding wasn't so bad after all. Maybe I was just making too much of it. God, I didn't even want to think about being so empty inside. Nothing was making any sense to me. I never wanted to be pregnant again, but I had to know I could be. And what if I lost all interest in sex? Would I age like the picture of Dorian Gray[1] in the next few years?

Finally I pulled my thoughts together and managed to speak. . . .

"Well, with planning I can pretty well cope with what is going on," I said. "Maybe we could go this route next year, if this keeps up."

As I sit here tonight, writing this, I find that the time that followed is not very clear in my mind. I can remember my doctor telling me to feel free to get a second opinion. It was almost as if I were a criminal being informed of my rights to one phone call. And yet I do trust my doctor.

There is no doubt in his mind that I need the hysterectomy and that it would be better to do it now than to risk emergency surgery at a time when I would feel pressed. And he is not trying to push me into a decision. He urged me to think about it—talk it over at home—and call his office to schedule surgery if and when I am ready.

And so I feel unbelievably numb tonight. I am trying to deal with so much information—and yet

---

[1] *The Picture of Dorian Gray* is a novel written by Oscar Wilde in 1891, in which the main character, Dorian Gray, remains unchanged through the years while his picture ages.

not enough information. The doctor said I would go on estrogen therapy if they removed my ovaries. I have read so many frightening things about the use of hormones. Will I get fat? Or grow a beard?

What about the weeks of taking it easy at home after the surgery? I am a single parent—and there are five kids in this family. Who can help? Will they resent this? Can they understand? Where do I turn for help? Where is the information? Am I the only woman nutty enough to have these fears about something which my doctor considers so routine?

Others

One of the best things about being busy and having lots of people to take care of is that you cannot spend all of your life trying to make decisions. When life is so daily, you find yourself coping.

And so I decided to have a hysterectomy. I didn't seek another opinion because I don't know any doctor whom I trust as much as I do my own. Besides, I really don't have enough information on which to base judgments of my own. And I don't have time to get a medical education.

When I called my doctor's office to say that I would go ahead with surgery, I was told that I should plan for some time after the third week in July. I felt satisfied with that because it gave me time to plan.

But something disturbing happened today. Actually, it made me more comfortable with my decision to have the hysterectomy.

I was in a workshop with about ten people, male and female, participating in the discussion. As the time drew near for us to take a break, I felt that familiar, warm, gushing sensation. Although I had used two fresh napkins only an hour earlier, I had the feeling that they would not be adequate. I was right. When I stood up—ever so carefully—blood ran down my leg. There was blood on the chair.

Some of the people in the group were able to deal with this and were even able to help me. But others were obviously embarrassed. One of the women did not return when we gathered together to complete our workshop.

This incident had brought back memories of other times when my problem created problems for others. I realize that I cannot allow this to go on. I am not a hermit. If I want to struggle along, this is one thing. But I feel I must consider how other people react.

As I drove home today, I knew that my decision was the only one I could make. It hasn't helped me feel less afraid or less anxious, but it has helped me feel more responsible. I am doing the best thing that I can do.

July 3, 1973

Time has run out. I had a phone call from my doctor today. He told me that there was an unexpected opening and that surgery could be scheduled for Thursday, July 12. Earlier we had talked about the third week in July. Now I am faced with a specific date, even sooner than I thought. What's the matter with me? There is a smooth, well-established procedure for me to follow. My mind is made up, isn't it?

All I need to do is report to the medical center within a few days and enter my medical history into the computer. Then I enter the hospital on July 11 and prepare for surgery. Everything is going to be just fine.

It struck me that I would be entering the hospital on what would have been my parents' forty-eighth wedding anniversary—only Daddy had died in January. So it seemed very important to remember to contact Mother and be supportive of her at this time. Good heavens, Mother had a hysterectomy at a private hospital when I was a little kid. I remember being pretty horrified by the scar. I sure don't need to remember that right now.

What about my own kids? They are all set, either visiting their dad or already on their own.

My job is under control. I'm not working for the summer. All seems clear on the job front.

What isn't resolved is the whole business of my fears and anxieties. I've tried really hard not to dwell on some of the fears I have, but they are all there just the same. I just don't want to lose an important part of my body. Even though I know that I do not want to bear another child, I need to know that I am able to do that. Not having that ability means that I am really over the hill—on my way to being old. I think I will even miss my menstrual periods, because they signal to me that all is well.

And if all is not well? What will happen—

especially if they remove my ovaries—and it seems as though they will? How much sooner will I grow older? Will any man want to make love to me—an aging female who has lost the capacity to reproduce? Males are raised to feel important because they have the capacity to impregnate a female. If I don't even have that capacity, will I ever attract a male?

And the mention of estrogen therapy, as hopeful as that sounds, has its own horrors. Who can help me deal with this?

What about the scar? I don't expect to model bikini bathing suits, but I like to think that I could continue to feel good about my body. No one has talked to me about the location or size of the incision.

Worst of all is the fear that I might not even make it out of the operating room. I can still hear my mother and my aunt discussing a childhood friend who died in her late thirties. She died on the operating table—it was a clot. "How awful. Poor Anna. Poor Anna's children."

And there was a forty-four year old woman in my community who died a few years ago right after surgery. The word that got out was, "When they cut her open she was so full of cancer that they sewed her right up again, and she died a day or two later."

These are my fears . . . and they are real.

I'd like to see my kids grow into adulthood. I'd like to fix up our home, now that I have a little more in the way of resources. I'd like to challenge myself to greater growth.

As I write this, I feel very afraid and very alone. I cannot dump this emotional load on my children. Most of my friends would not want to discuss this—perhaps they have their fears, too. When I have tried to talk about it, people brush me off with the comment that I am very healthy. Or they point out what a good doctor I have or what a good medical center we have. These things are true, and the percentage of failure may be small. But what if I am that statistic?

SURGERY

July 11, 1973

I came into the hospital today, and as usual, I really like it here. I have always liked being in hospitals, and my experiences have been good.

I have the room to myself now, but I will probably have a roommate soon. I brought in my typewriter and lots of books to read. It is so peaceful here. I don't have to shop or cook or do any laundry. And I can watch anything I want to on the television I've rented. This is great.

On Monday I fed my medical history into the computer. This computer then produces a very long and detailed printout which is available to the people who are responsible for my care.

Several things are happening to me—or have happened—or will happen. I wish I had had a little more preparation for this before I entered the hospital. Most of my other stays have been to have babies, and the procedure for surgery is different. A very fine young woman, who is a second year med student, came in to discuss my medical history. She was very thorough. This made me feel good—like she really cared. She was also warm and attentive, and I found myself pouring out all of my fears and anxieties to her. She didn't think that they were foolish—or that I was being unnecessarily mistrustful. She listened and encouraged me to say everything I needed to say. I felt as though a tremendous burden had been lifted from my shoulders.

She was very reassuring and gave me some information which I had not had before. Earlier in the day, a nurse asked me if I was going to have a vaginal or abdominal hysterectomy. I felt pretty stupid because I didn't even know about vaginal hysterectomies.

Ms. White explained to me that I would be having an abdominal hysterectomy. Because there was a high probability that my ovaries would be removed, the vaginal hysterectomy would not be practical. We also discussed my having my appendix removed and agreed that this was a wise decision. She calmed my fears by showing me where the incision would be made and reassured me that it would not be noticeable at all after awhile.

She began to sketch on a pad of paper, and as she shared information with me, I began to gain the confidence to ask questions. Now this hysterectomy was getting interesting. She made a diagram of how my vagina would be closed off. For the first time, I was beginning to understand what was going to happen.

Earlier this evening, Ms. White and I had another experience together. Even though I had had a pelvic examination, I was taken upstairs one flight, on a stretcher, where a resident supervised her while she did a pelvic examination on me. I suspect it was her first—at least her first on someone with my condition. I really didn't mind, but I wish everyone had been more honest about it. I value this medical center because it is a teaching hospital. And I really cared about this young woman. I am thrilled that she is becoming a doctor. She could have practiced on me all evening if it would have helped. I felt I was a member of the team, and I wish someone had recognized that.

This brings me to another issue. It is so nice when a member of the health care team says, "Hello, I'm so-and-so and my job is to do such-and-such." Some people do that, but it doesn't seem to be a uniform policy. This makes a tremendous difference. No one likes mystery people around at a time like this.

Also, I think that everyone who works in a hospital has the human right to be recognized and have their work valued. No one should have to work in the shadows. The people who come in to clean the room, change the water, and bring tissues can make a difference in how you feel.

My food tasted good at lunch and dinner. I won't be able to eat or drink anything else for awhile. But I look forward to choosing my meals again—from the menus you get a day ahead of time. Such luxury!

I have a roommate now. She seems to be about my age and is from a town near mine. She is having a D & C in the morning. It will be good to have company.

A Week in My Life

It's Wednesday night, and I am going home tomorrow.

So much has happened this past week. The night before surgery, my roommate and I enjoyed magnificent backrubs from one of the nurses. We chatted as we each ate two plain crackers and drank our glasses of orange juice. This was to be the last food I would see for five days. My doctor is a firm believer in no food until they hear bowel sounds.

I got so caught up in visiting that I forgot to go down the hall and phone Mother. It would have been her forty-eighth wedding anniversary. By the time I remembered it, I was all hooked up into intravenous apparatus. It wasn't usually possible to have a phone in the room, but they put one in so I could call her.

A lot of X-rays and other tests are necessary when you have surgery. I never learned about the results. I suppose I should feel all right about that since I guess everything was OK. But I still believe that payment for the tests entitled me to some indication of the results.

A very nice thing happened. I was wearing a POW bracelet (a bracelet worn by many U.S. citizens during the war in Viet Nam to protest the keeping of American military personnel as prisoners of war) and did not want it removed. I felt sure it was fruitless to mention this—but I did. The nurse looked at me for a minute and then said, "OK. I think we can leave it on. I'll tape it good." It was a great relief to me. A small thing, to be sure. But it helped my morale.

After all the preparations were made, it was just a matter of waiting for an opening in one of the operating rooms. I am sure there must be a reason that a schedule cannot be made out ahead of time. There was some indication that I might not even get into an operating room that day. This situation tended to increase my feeling of anxiety. Finally, however, my turn came at about two o'clock in the afternoon.

I now know how little had been explained to me in terms of what would be happening in surgery. For example, although I was aware that I would not be having general anesthesia, I did not have an understanding of what the procedure would be. I was unaware that there would be a frame screening my face from the rest of my body. And I did not know all the people in the room. I didn't need to know their names, but I would have been more comfortable if I had had a grasp of the roles that were being played by the various members of the team.

I dozed a good bit of the time. On two occasions I experienced discomfort that was sufficient to cause me to say something about it. I recall that I sensed a flurry of activity at that time. The anesthesiologist placed a mask over my mouth and nose and repeated to me, "Breathe, Kitten. Breathe!"

It was later explained to me that the discomfort I experienced was due to disturbance of my large intestine, once during exploratory work preceding surgery and once while they were removing my appendix.

I was returned directly to my room. I remember asking for something to ease the pain but was told I couldn't have anything. I insisted on seeing my doctor. He came to my bed and explained to me that I would be given medication as soon as my vital signs were normal. I was able to accept that.

My younger daughter came to visit me during this recovery time which I think was unfortunate because I upset her. I was dazed and incoherent, and she said I "looked green."

If I had it to do over again, I would suggest that my family members phone in for a report but not come to visit until the immediate recovery period was over.

By Friday morning I was sitting up in a chair while the nurse made my bed. Each day my mobility increased. I stayed on IV for several days and simply pulled it with me wherever I went.

Once the nurses asked me to go up to the next floor and talk with a woman who was in a situation similar to mine. She was about my age, divorced, and had several children. She hadn't had her hysterectomy yet and was experiencing many of the fears that I had. I think it really helped her to see me up and about, feeling quite positive so soon after surgery. I know it helped me to realize that I was not the only woman with these feelings.

Once my stitches were removed and I was no longer on IV, I was able to take a shower and shampoo my hair. I got on the scale and saw that I had lost seven pounds. Happiness!

I've had two more roommates during this week. One of the problems is a lack of privacy to talk with your doctor. Of course they pull the curtain around you, but voices can still be heard. I was anxious to discuss matters involving future sexual activity, and I found this difficult to do with a roommate present.

Another problem can be the issue of smoking. None of my roommates smoked, but their guests did. As a nonsmoker, I still haven't managed to be able to ask others not to smoke.

The visiting hours are very generous. Having friends and family drop in most any time avoids crowding everyone in at once. But there were times when I needed to doze and couldn't. Dozing during the day seems to be an important part of recovery. I think I am going to miss the security of the daily routine here. Each day starts early. I like a good breakfast and a chance to wash and change into a fresh johnny while my bed is being made. And the wonderful backrub that ends each day!

My doctor met with my son yesterday. He knows that it is up to the children to see that I follow his carefully prescribed instructions for my convalescence at home. He told my son not to hesitate to call him if he thought I was overdoing it. I think this will help the children feel more involved in my care once I get home. It seems strange to be leaving the hospital tomorrow without a baby . . . to be going home alone.

Good to be Home

I have been home for several days now. As I anticipated, I had some adjustments to make. The hospital insulates you from some of the realities of life, giving you a chance to get your physical self straightened out. Right now I feel tired. Even though the children are cooperating fully, I find that I am just doing more taking care of myself than I did a few days ago.

I have called the doctor's office twice. One time I made an appointment for my six weeks checkup. Another time I was concerned about my incision. It seemed red and was a little painful. The nurse told me to use hot soaks. That helped. Some of the worries are over. I didn't die in surgery. My scar isn't half bad, even now, and I am assured that it will fade in time. I feel quite attractive, and I am very much interested in sex.

I know I still have some things to work out. I was very much aware of not having a period when it was due. Actually, I was reminded of it because I felt a pulsating in my vagina, exactly the feeling I always had on the first day of my period. When I checked the calendar, I saw that my period probably would have started that day. I still feel concern about the fact that my ovaries were removed. I will be taking a tablet called Premarin the first twenty-five days of each month. (This is a synthetic estrogen preparation.) I should read more about the pros and cons of hormone therapy.

The hardest part about not being able to get pregnant again is that it is a sudden and definite end, psychologically, to an important period in my life. It will take time for me to work this through and accept it.

A WAY TO GROW

August 24, 1973

It has now been six weeks and one day since a hysterectomy was performed on me. I had a checkup today and the doctor is satisfied that everything is perfect. And as far as sexual activity is concerned, all systems are go.

My only other questions pertained to the timing of monthly self-examinations of my breasts and whether or not I needed annual checkups any longer. He suggested that I select a date each month that would be easiest for me to remember and examine my breasts regularly on that date.

It would be important for me to have a regular checkup each year. A Pap smear would still be done. And it would be wise, for the sake of my general health, to be examined.

During the six weeks since surgery, I had a lot of time to think about my situation. I decided that some kind of accurate and sensitive material should be made available to those women who wanted to know more about what was happening. I wanted to be a part of preparing such material, but I knew I needed help with the medical information. I summoned up my courage.

"You know, when I was in the hospital, I was given some printed material which said there was some information on hysterectomy available and that anyone interested should ask the nurse for it. I did ask, but no one knew what I was referring to. They checked around, but no material was ever found. Do you know what it is?"

"No," he answered thoughtfully. "I don't know what they were referring to."

"Well, I've done a little investigating. There doesn't seem to be much of anything available which can help a woman learn more about this surgery. I was thinking of writing an article or short book in consultation with a doctor. What do you think about that?"

"Oh, we do have a book here. Didn't you get a copy?"

"No, I didn't."

He left the room and returned shortly with a brief pamphlet. It was very disappointing, to say the least. The information was superficial. The copy was illustrated with foolish little cartoons. They reminded me of newspaper cartoons which depict men and women in stereotypic roles, ridiculing one another. I thanked him but realized that he hadn't really understood what I was talking about.

Today seemed to put a period and an exclamation mark at the end of this experience. I know that I must use caution for quite some time. I won't lift and carry heavy things. And I will try to get enough rest and watch my diet.

Perhaps my most important challenge is to begin to think of myself in a new way. I truly have become a different person by going through this experience. My desire to assume more responsibility for my body and what happens in connection with it has grown to a desire to assume responsibility for everything about myself. It is exciting!

Summer, 1974—

This has been a strange, strange summer. The kids are growing up and working away from home.

Last summer I saw this coming. I remember thinking that the most difficult thing about the hysterectomy was that it put a sudden and definite end to an important period in my life. I knew that it would take time for me to work through and accept the fact that childbearing was over—and childrearing was a role I would be phasing out with certainty. No replacements would ever come along. No fantasies were left.

I recall a time, years ago, when the children were still quite small. For reasons I can no longer remember, every child was absent from home for a period of twenty-four hours at the same time! I planned to get a great deal of work done in a quiet, peaceful house. To my amazement, I accomplished nothing. I simply could not function in that house alone. I wandered around aimlessly. I didn't feel like watching television. I couldn't read. And it was impossible for me to organize myself to start work on any of the dozen projects I had in mind. I was a mother—and a mother needs kids around in order to do her thing.

But this is getting to be less and less true. Oh, I still enjoy my children. I am still their mother—very much so. But I am much more able to live for myself now. I see myself as a person who has a great deal to contribute to young children and their families. I see myself as a woman who recognizes her strengths and vulnerabilities—a woman who is able to be responsible for herself. I am spending a lot of energy planning for the exciting years I have yet to live. It has worked out for me, but I cannot help but feel that the experience could have been more positive. I needed more knowledge. I needed more support. I needed to feel that I had been an informed decision maker. I do not want life to happen to me. I want to be able to make choices, and I feel sure there are other women who feel this way.

The future is filled with unknowns for every human being. I have learned that life's changes, like the seasons, are often dramatic—yet predictable. Knowing that I have the ability to assume responsibility for myself in this pattern has given me a good feeling about myself. I don't have to depend on a male figure. I am enjoying my sense of new freedom.

TAKING CHARGE
OF YOUR OWN BODY

As an informed person, you should be better able to ask questions, to participate in making decisions, and to understand the rationale behind your own health care. The following chapters are included to help you with that process.

"Participating in the Decision" provides information that will increase your understanding of the anatomy and physiology of your reproductive system, of the hormones that control its function, and of some of the conditions which *may* necessitate surgery. The examination and diagnostic tests are included to help you understand how your physician makes a diagnosis and recommendations. A knowledge of procedures, therapies, alternatives to and results of hysterectomy can correct misinformation and alleviate unjustified fears and concerns.

An explanation of hospital policy and surgical procedure is provided in the second chapter, "Your Hospital Stay: Admission to Discharge." Its purpose is to help you understand what is happening during this time.

"You! A Member of Your Health Team" is included to help you see that you not only have rights but also responsibilities for your own health. This may mean that you have to psych yourself up to act differently than you have in the past. It is probable that many doctors—especially men—will find it difficult to relate to an assertive female patient who wants to take responsibility for her own health care decisions. This simply means that you try harder!

Some important insights and some specific suggestions of things which all adults can do right now to help children grow up more free of sex role stereotypes can be found in "Kiss Cinderella Goodbye."

And a new beginning for all of us is the final chapter, "Today is the First Day. . . ." Will you act to start taking care of that very important person who is you? As two women who care about ourselves, we care about you—and we hope you will find your own special way to "becoming."

Participating in the Decision

When faced with the decision of hysterectomy what are some of the things which would be helpful to know? When faced with the reality of this surgery—and the hospital stay—what information should you have? The first two chapters in this section will try to provide some of this information.

We all make decisions every day. Some of them are fairly simple, with no particularly significant long-range implications. What shall I prepare for dinner tonight? Which TV program shall I watch? Other decisions are more involved, more difficult and have definite long-range implications. Shall I buy a new car? Should I purchase a home? How should I invest my money? And maybe for you now, should I have that hysterectomy?

For some women, because of the diagnosis or because of such factors as age, completed childbearing, pain or bleeding, the decision may be easy. They will feel that their doctor's recommendation to have a hysterectomy is the right one and will be in agreement from the beginning. This is the decision they sought. For others the recommendation may be disturbing and threatening. It may have come as a surprise; or it may be difficult to accept even though it was suspected. For this group the most helpful thing might be to seek information and take an objective look at the situation in order to make a realistic decision.

Reproductive function and any related disturbances are linked with social and emotional factors during every phase of a woman's life. Each phase involves feelings about femininity and childbearing ability. These feelings, which become paramount in making or accepting a decision about any procedure that interrupts them, are one reason why a decision concerning hysterectomy can be so difficult.

Many gynecologists feel the decision should be theirs; patients go to them because of their knowledge and expertise and because they are best qualified to judge. From a medical viewpoint this is so. But since this decision affects the basic symbol of femininity to a woman—her uterus—time to consider what the effects will be and to participate in the final decision are important.

Several steps are involved if you are faced with making this particular decision: defining the problem, analyzing the information you have, considering the alternatives and exploring them with others. Hopefully, you have already decided to have regular gynecological examinations so that any problems can be identified and treated promptly. Any irregular bleeding, changes in normal menstrual patterns, or pain should alert you to a possible problem and send you to your physician before the next appointment is due. Defining your problem or making a diagnosis may be just a matter of a physical examination or it may involve laboratory and diagnostic tests. This may take time. Your physician bases his recommendations on the findings of your examination and the results of any tests done, to assist you in making your decision.

Going through the steps of the decision-making process will help you sort things out and look at the situation in a more realistic and informed way. First, write down the medical facts and put them together with your feelings, preferences, home and family situation and any other factors important to you. A critical step in decision making is being sure you have correct information. Next, consider the alternatives: If I choose alternative *A* what will be the outcome? If I choose *B* what will be the result? Most solutions have both positive and negative aspects. Make a list of the alternatives by writing down what you see as the choices and outcomes. The final decision is, ultimately, yours alone. However, exploring alternatives with your physician and health professionals will add correct medical information; exploring them with family and those closest to you may help with the less tangible factors.

It is our hope that being better informed will help you to ask questions, to participate in the decision for surgery and to be comfortable and secure with that decision once it is made.

THE REPRODUCTIVE SYSTEM
AND ITS FUNCTIONS

    The female reproductive system is composed of the external genitalia (vulva and vagina) and the internal organs (uterus, tubes and ovaries). The vulva consists of the labia, which are two raised folds of tissue covering the clitoris, a small erectile organ, and the urinary meatus, through which urine is passed. The vaginal opening is below the meatus and above the rectum. There are two small glands on either side of the vagina which secrete mucous for lubrication during intercourse. The vaginal canal is about 4 inches long and leads up to the uterus. The lower portion of the uterus, which extends into the vagina, is the cervix. Those of you who have had babies will remember this as the portion which dilates during labor. Above the cervix is the body of the uterus, situated between the bladder and rectum. It is a small organ normally about 3 inches long and 2 inches wide. Extending outward from the uterus are the Fallopian tubes, about four inches long. Just below the open end of each tube lie the ovaries, approximately ½ by 1 inch in size. The diagram shows the relationship of these organs.

    The uterus plays a central role in a woman's feelings about her femininity: it is a uniquely female organ. At the time of puberty, the pituitary gland releases hormones which stimulate the ovaries to produce estrogen and progesterone. These are essential hormones in female physiology and are responsible for breast development, sexual hair growth and maturity of female sex organs. Under the influence of estrogen

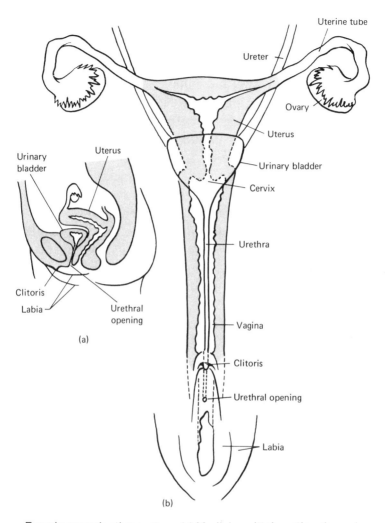

Female reproductive system. (a) Medial sagittal section through female pelvis, showing reproductive organs. (b) Diagrammatic frontal view of reproductive organs. Uterus and vagina are shown in section; lower end of vagina is shown in transparency behind external sex organs. (From Dexter M. Easton, *Mechanisms of Body Functions,* © 1974 by Prentice-Hall, Inc.; p. 452. Reprinted by permission of Prentice-Hall, Inc.)

and progesterone, the lining of the uterus thickens. If fertilization does not occur, the lining is not needed and is shed from the uterus during menstruation. If fertilization does occur, these hormones are responsible for preparing the uterus to receive the egg and for changes necessary to provide the environment for the development and nurturing of the unborn baby. Produced during each menstrual cycle and throughout pregnancy, these two hormones are what some women feel to be the essence of their femaleness.

The physiological decrease in the production of estrogen and progesterone is gradual and occurs in most women between forty-five and fifty-five years of age. As hormone levels decrease, ovarian and uterine changes gradually occur. The word menopause means cessation of menstruation. During this time, the interval between periods becomes longer, and the flow usually decreases in amount. Some women experience a wide variety of symptoms at menopause. One of the most common is the hot flash resulting from vasomotor (vessel) changes. Another is a dryness or itching of the vagina as tissue changes occur. Other symptoms that may be experienced by some women are headaches, weight gain, nervousness, heart palpitation, difficulty sleeping, or feelings of uselessness or depression. For the majority of women these symptoms, while annoying, are not severe enough to require medical treatment. They are normal and they are temporary. By the time most women have reached the mid-forties they have heard so many tales about the menopause that they have trouble separating fact from fiction. The fact is that only one out of four women will have symptoms severe enough to need treatment of any kind. As surgical procedures are discussed, remember: hormones are produced by the ovaries, so removal of the uterus alone has no effect on hormone levels. The symptoms mentioned previously are experienced only during physiological menopause or when both ovaries are completely removed.

HOW THE PHYSICIAN
MAKES A DIAGNOSIS

The Pelvic Examination

As previously mentioned, the procedures upon which your physician bases a diagnosis include the pelvic examination and diagnostic tests. Most or maybe even all of you have had a pelvic examination, but perhaps only a few of you know just what was being done or why. A brief review might be helpful. The examination consists of two main parts: the speculum examination and the manual examination. A speculum is a metal or plastic instrument with two rounded blades that is inserted into the vagina and then opened so the vaginal walls and cervix can be seen. They are observed for color, condition of tissue, and the presence of any abnormalities. At this time secretions can be obtained from the cervix for a Pap smear or for other laboratory tests, including those for infection or for estrogen level. This is the reason for not douching or using any vaginal creams or medications twenty-four hours prior to the examination. They interfere with the normal secretions and affect the test being done.

The manual examination is done to feel the cervix, body of the uterus, ovaries and adjacent structures. With two fingers in the vagina and one hand on the abdomen, the examiner can feel the uterus between the two hands and examine it for size, shape, irregularities or tenderness. By moving the hands to the right and left sides, he or she can examine the ovaries in the same way. During this examination you should only feel pressure; in the absence of pathology it should not be painful.

If you do experience tenderness or pain, be sure to let your physician know. This information is helpful in making a diagnosis. Remember, pain occurs or is made worse by fear and tension. Knowledge of the procedure and relaxation are the keys to alleviating this anxiety. Breathing slowly and rhythmically through the mouth helps relax abdominal muscles. Keeping your eyes open and focusing on some object in the room helps to concentrate on maintaining this breathing. These are the same techniques many of you used during labor, and they work beautifully during examinations too. A rectal examination usually concludes the pelvic examination. Although uncomfortable for the patient, it is valuable to feel the uterus from another perspective and to confirm the findings of the vaginal examination.

If your physician has any questions based on your history or the pelvic examination, further diagnostic tests might well be ordered. Some of the more common ones are included here to familiarize you with them. Since practice varies, be sure to clarify details with your own physician and/or his nurse.

Diagnostic Tests

OF THE CERVIX

Probably the first and most common test is the Pap smear. Named for Dr. Papanicolaou who first described it, the procedure involves obtaining cells from the cervix and "smearing" them on a slide for microscopic study. It is painless and done while the speculum is in place. You won't even be aware of it. If there is any question about the appearance of the cells on the Pap smear, a colposcopy might be ordered.

Colposcopy is a more comprehensive method of visualizing the cervix than that performed with a speculum alone. Done with a colposcope, a magnifying instrument with a bright light that is focused through the speculum, the entire cervix can be scanned to examine tissue and blood vessels and to determine if any irregularities or lesions are present. The procedure is the same as that of the speculum examination. It is not painful and requires only a few minutes.

If additional cells or tissue are needed for further microscopic study, a biopsy (obtaining bits of tissue) can be done during the colposcopic examination. These are then examined by a pathologist for diagnosis.

OF THE ENDOMETRIUM

The endometrium, lining of the uterus, can be evaluated by inserting an instrument through the os, or opening of the cervix, to obtain a tissue specimen. This sometimes causes a momentary cramp. It is the same sensation as when an intrauterine device is inserted and so may be familiar to some of you. Endometrial biopsies are evaluated by the

45

pathologist for any abnormalities and yield valuable diagnostic information. They are often done to determine the presence or absence of ovulation in infertility problems; the levels of estrogen and progesterone and their effect on development of the lining; and the presence of infection, lesions or tissue changes due to causes ranging from the effects of contraceptive pills to malignancy. Depending on the results of these or other tests, the physician is better able to confirm whether changes are within normal limits or, if not, to make a diagnosis. All of these tests are office procedures. They do not require any special preparation or anesthesia and take only a few minutes to perform.

POSSIBLE SURGICAL PROCEDURES

Dilatation and Curettage

Commonly known as a D & C, this is by far the most common gynecological procedure. It is both diagnostic and therapeutic and can be performed by suction curettage in the physician's office or as a surgical procedure under anesthesia in the hospital.

A D & C is done as a diagnostic procedure to obtain endometrial tissue for the same reasons the biopsy was done. The advantage of curettage is that more representative tissue samples from a variety of areas can be obtained and given to the pathologist for study. A D & C is *therapeutic* when performed to treat a bleeding problem or to remove the contents of the uterus. D & C's are also performed for *incomplete* or therapeutic abortions, and for correction of irregular bleeding patterns. Abortions are termed incomplete when all tissue from the pregnancy is not expelled spontaneously; some of it is retained in the uterus and a D & C is used to fully empty the uterus. A D & C may also be done for a therapeutic or elective abortion, that is, one chosen to eliminate an unwanted pregnancy. Some conditions lend themselves readily to the "suction" method, but if the physician needs to do a more thorough and complete examination than can be done in the office, the surgical procedure under anesthesia will be preferable.

Hysterectomy

On few topics is there more misinformation and more unjustified fear and anxiety than on that of hysterectomy alone or hysterectomy plus removal of the tubes and ovaries.

Hysterectomy is feared by some women because they feel there will be no further enjoyment of sexual relations, that they will gain weight, their skin will look "old" and wrinkled, that hair growth or distribution will change. Fear of psychological change becoming forgetful, getting depressed, or even losing one's mind—is common. These are not the direct result of removal of the uterus and should not influence your decision. They are discussed further in the last chapter.

On the other hand, for some women the function of the uterus is unimportant. A menstrual period is indeed the monthly "curse." The childbearing process may be completed, or children may not be desired. Pain and/or bleeding may have become intolerable. For these women, the uterus is readily dispensible.

Hysterectomy means removal of the uterus. Removal of the entire uterus is a total hysterectomy. This may be accomplished abdominally or vaginally. Several factors are considered in determining which approach is best. For example, tumors usually require an abdominal incision. They may be too large to be removed through the vagina and can be removed through the abdomen more easily. There may be adhesions in the pelvis or problems with the ovaries or tubes, or your physician may want to inspect other organs in the abdomen. In these instances an abdominal approach would be used.

Sometimes the uterus is displaced downward into the vagina (a prolapse), or the vaginal walls become relaxed, causing the bladder or the rectum to protrude into the vagina (a cystocele or a rectocele). In these situations removing the uterus vaginally and repairing the vaginal walls at the same time may be the best procedure.

Oophorectomy

Oophorectomy means removal of the ovaries. This must be accomplished through an abdominal incision. Ovaries are removed for such conditions as endometriosis, cysts or tumors. In addition, age may be a determining factor. In pre-menopausal women many physicians will try to preserve one or even part of one ovary to maintain estrogen production.

Remember that the ovaries continue to produce hormones whether the uterus is present or not. Therefore, a hysterectomy does not affect hormone levels unless the ovaries are both completely removed. Complete removal of both ovaries produces a surgical menopause. One ovary will continue to produce hormones even if the rest of the reproductive organs are removed, but should both ovaries need to be completely removed, the adrenal glands do produce some estrogen which may be sufficient to eliminate or minimize any symptoms of menopause. If not, hormone replacement therapy might be considered. An oophorectomy is of major concern to many women who feel that physical and psychological changes will occur without estrogen. Estrogen replacement is an issue being discussed in the media as well as in the medical community. Therefore, some information is included here with the hope you will be aware and discuss this with your physician before surgery so your treatment will be understood.

THE HORMONE CONTROVERSY

Hormone therapy is controversial because there are so few controlled studies, fewer long-term studies and many unanswered questions. One reason for this is the fact that the life span has increased so markedly in the last decades that only recently has hormone therapy become a concern, and only fairly recently have hormones become available for prescription. With the increase in life span, many women are living beyond the menopausal years, so the need for hormone supplements has increased markedly. When life expectancy was about 50 years of age, it coincided with the cessation of hormone production. This is no longer true, as many women have a third of their lives beyond the menopausal years. Because the medical profession is continually conducting research into both the physical and emotional aspects of the menopause, knowledge about hormones is advancing.[1]

Medical science has determined that estrogen replacement is valuable in women with symptoms specific to lack of estrogen. For example, hot flashes resulting from vasomotor instability respond to estrogen. Dryness and itching of the vagina are caused by a lack of estrogen, and the use of estrogen in pill form or as a vaginal cream will offer relief. Estrogen therapy can only ward off problems specifically associated with hormone deficiency.

Medical science also knows that estrogen therapy does not retard aging. It does not provide eternal youth. It does not make one look young or feel young, increase sex appeal or desire.

As with all drugs, the benefits of treatment must be weighed against the risks. For some symptoms the benefits are substantial. However, there remains much controversy

---

[1]Leon Speroff, et al., "The Estrogen Replacement Controversy," *Contemporary OB/GYN,* 8 (September 1976), 143.

over both the advantages and the hazards. Indeed, there is debate over the nature of the menopause itself, whether it be the result of physiological processes or oophorectomy.

Controversy arises over the use of estrogen to prevent osteoporosis (decrease in bone density from calcium loss); to prevent cardiovascular disease (high blood pressure, heart attacks, hardening of the arteries); or to relieve symptoms of nervousness, depression or insomnia.[2] There is a marked difference of opinion as to whether it is beneficial for these conditions. Another controversy arises over the use of estrogen therapy for women who undergo a normal physiological menopause versus those who undergo a surgical menopause. When the ovaries are removed before the onset of a natural menopause, there is an abrupt cessation of hormone production in contrast to the gradual decrease of a physiological menopause. Symptoms may be more exaggerated or severe, and therapy may be needed. At the present time the relationship between estrogen therapy and breast cancer is not clear, and a more thorough evaluation is needed. Self breast examination should be done by all women regularly, every month, so they will be familiar with their own bodies and able to detect changes. The majority of breast changes continue to be detected by women themselves. (See Resource section.)

Estrogen therapy may be contraindicated in women with high blood pressure, heart disease, liver disease or breast diseases. There is evidence that this hormone may

---

[2]Ronald Strickler, "The Climateric Woman: To Replace or Not Replace Estrogens," *Contemporary OB/GYN,* 8 (August 1976), 100.

advance these and other diseases, and only your physician can determine if this therapy would be safe.

One of the major concerns is the possibility that the prolonged use of estrogen predisposes or causes the development of cancer. Any number of studies have reported large numbers of women who have developed cancer of the lining of the uterus following estrogen therapy. Estrogen is a substance that produces growth the nature of which is still under study. Obviously the danger of uterine cancer is eliminated in women who have had hysterectomies, and many physicians feel safe in giving estrogen to this group.

The aim of hormonal therapy is to control symptoms as quickly as possible with as little medication as possible. Regular physician visits are necessary so that the proper dosage and regimen can be prescribed and adjusted according to symptoms. Vaginal smears can be taken for estrogen levels as a check of the effectiveness of therapy. Once started, some women will need to continue estrogen therapy indefinitely, while others may be able to have the dose decreased or the medication gradually withdrawn. Although this decision will be made by your physician, you should be informed about it and feel comfortable discussing it. The circumstances are so varied and there are such differences of opinion that only through discussion of the pros, cons, and alternatives can the best and safest decision be reached.[3]

---

[3]"Estrogen Therapy: the Dangerous Road to Shangri-La," *Consumer Reports,* 41:11 (November 1976), 642.

ALTERNATIVES TO SURGERY

For a number of years the question of unnecessary surgery in general and unnecessary hysterectomy in particular has been discussed. On September 21, 1975, the *New York Times Magazine* published an article stating that "more than 690,000 women will have hysterectomies in the United States in 1975—this will be the nation's second most frequently performed major operation—almost half of women over 40 will be advised to have hysterectomies and they will pay $400 million in gynecologist fees."[4]

As far back as 1971, Dr. Lawrence P. Williams in his book *How to Avoid Unnecessary Surgery* wrote that "hysterectomy ranks second after tonsillectomy in the number of unnecessary operations performed yearly."[5] Even *Ladies Home Journal* joined in with an article on the "Needless Hysterectomy" in March, 1976. As a result of such writings, the medical profession is concerned that patients will become suspicious when surgery is recommended, will decide against needed operations or will even neglect prompt diagnosis and treatment.

Patients become confused when deluged by books and articles with conflicting statistics and advice. How will

---

[4]*New York Times Magazine* (New York: The New York Times Company), *CXXIV* (Sunday, September 21, 1975).

[5]Lawrence P. Williams, *How to Avoid Unnecessary Surgery* (Los Angeles: Nash Publications, 1971), p. 134.

they know whether their recommended hysterectomy is really necessary, how will they find out, how will they make intelligent, responsible decisions?

An informed patient who asks thoughtful questions will create reciprocal respect. Keep your options open, question what you do not understand, seek information.

The following information on hysterectomies and alternatives will raise some issues and questions for you to pursue. For some, alternatives to hysterectomy are very viable choices; for others, removing the uterus is the only real solution.

In making your decision the major questions now become: What makes the surgery elective? What makes surgery necessary or even mandatory as a life-saving procedure? What, if any, are the alternatives to surgery?

Hysterectomy is elective if alternative methods of treatment, such as drug therapy, or a more conservative surgical procedure are possible, or if the symptoms of the condition are not threatening to the patient's life.

Although it is impossible to discuss all the conditions which might respond to alternative therapy, a few of the more common ones are included here to give you some idea of what is meant by alternative therapy and, more importantly, what questions to raise with your physician.

Uterine Bleeding

Because bleeding is a symptom and not a diagnosis, its cause must be determined. There are several irregular bleeding patterns related to hormone levels, ovulation, infections and tumors that may respond to drug therapy or a D & C. Sometimes bleeding occurs from blood diseases or endocrine problems and is not related to a uterine problem at all. It will cease with appropriate medical treatment. Abnormal bleeding can occur at any age and may last from a few hours to a few weeks. It can occur with or without pain or cramps. The most important first step with any unusual bleeding or pain is to see your physician for diagnosis. In so doing, remember that some conditions might be treated or controlled without surgery. Two of the more common ones are endometriosis and small myomas.

ENDOMETRIOSIS

Endometriosis is a condition in which endometrial tissue grows on organs or structures outside the uterus, commonly the ovaries and pelvic ligaments. The growth of this tissue depends on hormone stimulation during the menstrual cycle. Cysts may form, and with each cycle they increase in size. Depending on the location and severity of the disease, the age of the patient and desire for children, conservative surgery such as removing the cysts or hormone therapy to suppress ovulation may be successful. (Hormones increase during pregnancy, so the disease often goes into remission. If children are desired, it is safe to attempt pregnancy, and conservative therapy should be attempted.) Many times this condition will regress or be controlled by stopping ovarian activity.

BENIGN TUMORS

Uterine myomas (fibroids) are the most common benign tumors. They may be of any size and occur singly or multiply on the inner or outer surface of the uterus. Bleeding is the most common symptom, but if large enough, they may cause pressure on the bladder and/or bowel. Backache is common. Growth of myomas depends at least partly on hormone stimulation. Many will regress after menopause. If symptoms are not severe, careful observation may be all that's needed. A myomectomy, removal only of the myoma, may be tried if it is desirable to preserve the uterus and reproductive function. Methods of conservative treatment will depend on the size and location of the myoma and the amount of bleeding it causes.

Two Other Problems

INFECTIONS

Uterine infections generally occur when bacteria enter through the cervix and infect the endometrium. If untreated, they may spread to the tubes and ovaries. In the acute phase most infections are treated with antibiotics. However, some infections become chronic and recurrent. Pain is usually the dominant symptom. If the infection cannot be controlled with antibiotics and abscesses or masses result, surgery may be indicated. Sometimes conservative surgery will be successful.

UTERINE PROLAPSE

When there is relaxation of the vaginal walls, the uterus may protrude into the vagina, causing discomfort and pressure on the bladder or bowel. Although vaginal hysterectomy is a successful solution for the problem, the use of a pessary can be considered. Pessaries come in all shapes and sizes and can be fitted into the upper vagina to support the uterus and hold it in place.

Hysterectomy becomes necessary when:

> myomas become so large they interfere with other body organs (such as hindering bladder or bowel functions);
>
> a tumor is of the type that might become malignant if not removed;
>
> bleeding is so heavy that it cannot be controlled or so frequent that anemia results. It then becomes not only debilitating but life-threatening, and hysterectomy may be the only recourse. This is true regardless of the cause of the bleeding;
>
> a pathologic condition exists that cannot be treated otherwise. A prime example of this would be cancer. We know that certain cancers spread, and the only way to arrest spread is to remove the organ involved.

Earlier in this chapter, some factors, concerns and symptoms were mentioned which might be of sufficient import to influence your decision. Feelings about femininity, the aging process, body image, sexuality, social and marital happiness are all to be considered.

The last chapter contains more detail and offers some specific suggestions. Remember that neither physiological menopause nor surgical removal of the uterus need change you or your relationships with your husband, family, friends or society.

In summary, the alternatives to hysterectomy are

basically twofold: drug therapy and/or more conservative surgical procedures.

Remember, too, that symptoms of some benign conditions may bother one woman more than another. Only you can evaluate whether your symptoms affect your daily life and therefore your willingness to try alternative therapies.

And lastly, remember, in spite of what you read and hear, that hysterectomy is the only real solution to *some* problems. An open discussion with your physician is the obvious place to begin.

Some questions you might want to ask:

Is alternative therapy going to cure the problem?

If not, how long can I expect relief?

Is it possible, or safe, to become pregnant?

If I take medication or have conservative surgery now, will a hysterectomy be needed eventually anyway?

What are the chances of getting better/worse?

What are the risks or side effects of the alternative therapy?

It is only by exploring all your options that you can make a wise decision with which you feel secure.

Your Hospital Stay: Admission to Discharge

Surgery is always a major experience in the lives of patients and their families. From the moment your physician makes a diagnosis you may be faced with the decision of accepting surgery.

Surgery is almost always performed in a hospital. Although you may be aware that many wonderful things are done there, a hospital is still a place where one goes when seriously ill or in need of an operation. A hospital is still a place of unknowns: where one may lose freedom, control, and even identity. Surgery represents physical intervention, anesthesia, loss of a body part, fear of what will be found, fear of pain, fear of disfigurement or disability, even fear of death.

When confronted with the need for surgery and all its related experiences, a period of uncertainty, anxiety and stress is bound to ensue. Perhaps you wish you had a little more preparation for your hospital stay.

Every hospital has its own policies and procedures, every physician his or her own preferences, and every one of you is a different individual with your own needs and requirements. Still there are certain commonalities to having a hysterectomy.

Most of you will enter the hospital a day or two ahead of time. Before surgery, known as the preoperative period, a complete history, physical examination, laboratory tests and X-rays are required. So, too, is a "pre-op prep." This includes stopping all foods and fluids, shaving the surgical area, an enema, a douche, and medications.

For surgery, medications, intravenous infusions, going to the operating room and anesthesia are all part of the experience.

Following surgery, monitoring your physical condition, providing for your body's oxygen and nutrition requirements, keeping you comfortable and relieving pain will be of first priority.

Several things will indeed happen to you. This section cannot answer all the questions you will need to ask, but it may provide some new information and suggest some questions you might want to discuss with your doctor and other members of the health care team.

THE MEDICAL HISTORY

Some of you will feed your medical history into a computer in advance, and the printout will be available when you come to the hospital. Others of you will receive a questionnaire to complete before admission; still others will be interviewed before or at the time of admission. Regardless of method, a complete history of past and present illnesses and conditions is important. Surgery and anesthesia produce changes in the body, and you must be in the best possible condition to withstand these changes. Knowledge of your medical history enables the members of your health team to plan the best and safest care possible. Be as thorough and accurate in giving your medical history as you can. You may want to make some notes of significant dates and data in advance.

THE PHYSICAL EXAMINATION

Your present physical condition determines any special procedures you will need before, during, and after surgery. Any coexisting condition influences the management of your care. We live in two environments: the external one of heat and cold, plants and animals, sights and sounds; and the internal one of the human body, guided by its systems to maintain equilibrium. Your external environment, home, job, recreation, and economics influence your operative course. Internally you are operated by cells, constantly adapting to changes in body requirements, capable of growing and functioning as long as they are provided with oxygen and nutrition. A thorough physical examination plus information from laboratory tests will indicate whether all your "systems are go" and, if not, how to best plan for your care. This involves examination of eyes, ears, nose, and throat, heart and lungs, abdomen, extremities and pelvic organs. If you enter a "teaching hospital," both house staff (interns and residents) and students (medical and nursing) will be members of your health team. Although they are learners, you will find most of them thorough, up to date, and interested. They participate in your care under the direction of your physician. Dee Dee's experience was typical. Do not hesitate to ask them questions; most will welcome the opportunity to explain procedures and provide you with information.

Nutritional status is evaluated to ensure the best possible postsurgery recovery. When there is a protein deficiency, wounds heal slowly and there is a decreased resistance to infection. A lack of vitamin C slows wound healing. Dehydration (vomiting or diarrhea deplete fluids rapidly) denies cells the nutrition they need. Keep this in mind when we discuss the use of intravenous (IV) infusions and the fact that foods and fluids are discontinued twelve to twenty-four hours before surgery.

LABORATORY TESTS

Some of the more common laboratory tests are mentioned here. You may expect several of these.

A complete blood count (CBC) includes hemoglobin levels and a red blood cell count which measures how well the blood is being oxygenated. When blood is drawn from an arm vein, a sample is also collected for type and cross match.

This is so compatible blood can be reserved for you at the blood bank. Should you need blood replacement, it's reassuring to know it is ready.

No doubt all of you have provided a specimen for urinalysis before. Whenever the body is placed under stress the capacity of the kidney to function is of great significance. Urine testing is one method of determining kidney status before surgery as well as its ability to handle fluids during the postoperative period.

An electrocardiogram (EKG) is a record of the activity of the heart muscle. The ability to deliver adequate amounts of oxygen and nutrition to cells depends on the heart as a pump and the condition of blood vessels. By placing electrodes on selected skin areas your heart cycle can be recorded. Chest X-rays and a test for vital capacity will supply data on pulmonary function—the ability of your lungs to provide oxygen and get rid of carbon dioxide.

OTHER TESTS

Two other tests are often done prior to a hysterectomy. Since the uterus lies in such close proximity to the urinary system and the lower bowel, an intravenous pyelogram (IVP) and/or barium enema may be ordered. Both of these are X-ray tests. In an IVP a dye is injected into an arm vein. This is picked up by the kidneys and excreted through the ureters into the bladder, enabling visualization of these organs on X-ray. For a barium enema, barium is put into the bowel through a rectal tube for the same purpose. The worst part of these tests is having to lie on the cold, hard X-ray table for thirty minutes or more.

THE NIGHT BEFORE SURGERY

Several procedures are required before you go to the operating room—the so-called pre-op prep. These are usually done the night before surgery so that, once completed, you can get as much rest as possible.

Preparation of the skin decreases the possibility of the entrance of bacteria into the wound from the skin surface at the time of surgery. Shaving the area and cleansing with an antiseptic solution reduces bacteria and promotes healing, thereby minimizing the risk of infection.

Preparation of the bowel requires one or more enemas. The purpose is to empty the bowel as much as possible, to increase visibility of the operative site and to protect it from injury. It also lessens difficulty from constipation postoperatively and may even prevent some of those infamous "gas pains." Preparation of the vagina is done through douching with an antiseptic solution to reduce bacteria and cleanse the area of secretions.

Discontinuing foods and fluids allows the stomach and bowel to be empty at the time of surgery—preventing nausea and vomiting and reducing trauma. Your water pitcher will be removed so you won't forget. An intravenous solution may be started at this time to maintain adequate fluids in your system since you are not permitted to drink. Coughing and deep breathing exercises will be taught so you can practice ahead of time. They are essential after surgery to prevent chest congestion and promote good lung expansion. A rubber glove, balloon or mechanical respirator may be used to assist you.

A few questions you may want to ask: What time is surgery scheduled? Will I go to a recovery room? When shall I tell my family to come? Can they call for a report? Who? When?

Make a list of questions in advance. You'll feel more relaxed and rest better when everything is organized and anticipated ahead of time.

Once all these preparations are completed, you will be ready to settle down for the night. Although important, they can be tiring. Sedation will be ordered to ensure maximal rest. Do take the drug and try to have your environment as quiet and comfortable as possible to receive maximum effect from the medication. Little things you're used to—open window, pulled shades, extra blanket—can make a big difference.

THE MORNING OF SURGERY

A bath or shower will feel relaxing and assure maximum cleanliness. You'll be asked to wear a hospital "johnny"—to prevent damage or loss of your personal clothes.

Dentures and contact lenses might create a danger for you, especially if general anethesia is used, and should be removed. Likewise jewelry—if removed in the operating room it might get lost. Your room or the nurses station is a safer place. There can be exceptions, as with DeeDee's POW bracelet, which we mentioned earlier, so if you feel strongly about something, ask your nurse. All makeup must be removed to allow for observation of color during surgery. About an hour before surgery, preoperative medication will be given to relax and prepare you for anethesia. Afterwards you'll need to be in bed—it should make you feel drowsy and at ease. The side rails on your bed will be raised for your protection and as a reminder to stay in bed.

Transportation to the operating room is usually by stretcher. The surgical team—your surgeon, his or her assistants, the anesthesiologist, and the surgical nurses—will be ready for you, albeit hard to recognize behind the caps and masks. They will help you move to the operating table to receive your anesthesia. Then you will be draped in preparation for the operation.

ANESTHESIA

One of the most commonly expressed concerns over having surgery is about anesthesia. Anesthesia for a hysterectomy is of two main types: general or regional.

General anesthesia puts you to sleep. It is produced by inhalation (breathing gas) or by injection (a drug injected into the blood stream) and affects all the body systems. Regional anesthesia is produced by injecting a drug to block out all sensation or feeling in the operative area. It affects only the designated region so you will be awake but will feel no pain. For a hysterectomy this will be a "spinal." Contrary to what you may have heard, spinal anesthesia is safe and provides excellent relaxation of the structures in the anesthetized area. And you'll probably nap during this time as DeeDee did. Fears and anxieties are commonly associated with anesthesia —a fear of going to sleep or a fear of being awake, a fear of "the mask" or of "the needle." The best remedy for these fears is a knowledge of what you will receive and why, what will be done and how you will feel. It is common practice for the anesthetist to visit the day before surgery. Anesthesia should be thoroughly discussed with him. If this is not the policy at your hospital, ask the nurse to explain it to you. Or ask both so you really do understand.

AFTER SURGERY

Following your hysterectomy, you may be returned to your room or to a recovery room. In either case certain procedures are carried out to ensure your optimal recovery. There are three phases to this recovery: (1) three or four days until metabolic and tissue changes return to normal, (2) four days to a week while other systems return to normal, and (3) a recuperative phase when strength returns.

Blood pressure, pulse and respiration will be checked frequently—as often as every ten or fifteen minutes. Commonly known as vital signs, they are just that, because they provide vital information as to your condition—how your body systems are responding to your surgery and anesthesia. Fluctuations up or down give information upon which to base your care. DeeDee requested medication and was told to wait until vital signs were stable. This may be hard to do—but the signs are so "vital" and are so easily altered by drugs that, for your safety, you may be asked to wait.

Remember the coughing and deep breathing exercises? They will be started now. Here are a couple of helpful hints:

If you had vaginal surgery, cross your legs at the ankles so you won't feel as though "everything is falling out." If you had abdominal surgery, support your incision with a pillow, pushing it in and down firmly.

Position is important to your comfort and to aid respiration and circulation. Nurses will assist with frequent turning; although it may hurt, changing position is essential. The side rails on your bed will be up for your safety; they are also very helpful when turning. Lying on your side with pillows for support reduces tension in the operative area and provides maximum comfort.

An intravenous infusion will provide fluid requirements until you can take them by mouth. Body fluid is constantly being lost and, for normal functions to occur, must be replaced. IVs are often continued for a few days. When bowel sounds can be heard, clear liquids are started and you will then advance to a regular diet. Remember that carbonated beverages tend to be "gassy," and juices or tea are more readily tolerated. One reason for waiting until bowel sounds are heard is to be sure GI (gastrointestinal) function is returning, thereby preventing the common complaint of "gas pains." If your mouth is dry, ask if you may have some ice chips, mouthwash or a small hard candy to suck.

What goes in must come out and a catheter (small tube into the bladder) allows urine to drain freely as it is produced. Because a hysterectomy necessitates surgery in close proximity to the bladder, swelling might occur and make voiding difficult. Once the swelling subsides (twenty-four to forty-eight hours) the catheter is usually removed. This also allows for a careful measurement of the amount of fluid you receive and the amount of urine you produce. Remember that equilibrium we are striving for?

Pain of some sort is almost an inevitable result of the mechanical trauma of surgery. Medication will be ordered for you which generally can be given safely every three to four hours as soon as your vital signs stabilize. For the first couple of days this is in injection form. When you are taking fluids, you may receive pain pills. Let the nurse know if you are having pain. Several things can be done to make you more comfortable. There's nothing to be gained by a "grin and bear it" attitude.

Some "problems" common to all major operations are mentioned here. Though not dangerous, they may be frightening or annoying.

Nausea, vomiting or hiccoughs
Pounding heart or palpitations
Shortness of breath
Flushing or sweating
Numbness or tingling
Feelings of anxiety or confusion

These usually represent your body's reactions to anesthesia and surgery and its efforts to adapt to changes in requirements. Let the nurse know if you experience any of them so she can assist with relief measures.

CONVALESCING

Ambulation (Walking)

The evening following surgery or the next morning you will be getting up. Naturally the first time will be the hardest. Do not try to get up alone. Your nurse will assist you. Early ambulation is essential to prevent complications. It promotes lung function, stimulates circulation, and starts you on the road to regaining muscle strength. Position changes will occur in stages, slowly, to minimize discomfort, and the nursing staff will assist and stay with you. With each successive period out of bed, strength and courage improve.

Rest

Regaining strength and becoming self-sufficient takes time. Do not overdo. Plan rest periods during the day and stick to them. Advise your family or other visitors so you won't be disturbed. As much as you might enjoy company, visiting can be very tiring and should be limited. Keep this in mind for the first few days at home as well.

Diet

High protein and iron rich foods help to heal and to rebuild. Eat meat, eggs, milk, poultry and fish if possible. Drinking a lot of fluid—about two quarts a day—prevents urinary problems and aids elimination. Fresh fruits and roughage help restore bowel function. Keep this in mind when you get home. If you need or desire a special diet, ask that the dietitian come and plan it with you.

Elimination

The best aid for proper elimination is dietary, but if bowel function is slow to return to what was normal for you, mild laxatives or stool softeners may be needed the first few days. As your food intake and ambulation increase, this will resolve.

Incision

Most dressings are removed a day or two after surgery. Sutures are removed before discharge. Most incisions heal without special treatment. Although they may look red and swollen and feel hard as the healing process takes place, this will subside within a few weeks until just a line of scar tissue remains.

Personal Activities

As soon as you feel up to it, a shower and shampoo will feel good. Getting out your cosmetics and other personal items adds to a sense of well-being. Resuming activities of daily living gives you added confidence. They become positive signs of progress. Add them slowly.

Going Home

Discharge planning is important and can make the transition from hospital to home smoother and easier. Will you have or need any help at home? What rearranging, if any, will be needed because of stairs, bathroom facilities, etc.? Will you need a special diet? Medicines? Treatments of any kind? What activities are allowed? Climbing stairs?

Lifting? Housework? Showers? Tub baths? What signs or symptoms are expected? When should you call the doctor? How about douches? Tampons? Sexual intercourse? Make a list of questions in advance so you won't forget to ask. You may feel well and your incision may look healed, but remember that it takes four to six weeks to heal on the inside. *Gradually* work up to normal activity. You will need to use caution for some time.

Discharge may put a period and an exclamation mark at the end of this experience, giving it an air of finality. A word about the way you may feel after you return home— feeling depressed, angry, threatened, changed, is normal. Some degree of depression almost always accompanies illness or surgery whether it be immediate or some time later. Inasmuch as it circumscribes your interests and activities and allows you to conserve energy, it is productive. You are proceeding from a stage of dependence to one of independence. You have lost a body organ.

Depression can be expressed in many ways: "I feel I could cry," "I'm not hungry," "I can't sleep"—or maybe you just feel lousy and can't figure out why.

Questions may arise: Was the surgery really necessary? Was it successful? Did I have cancer? Has my doctor told me the truth? These are important questions and need to be asked. Even if you've been told once, you may want to ask again to put your mind at ease.

Regaining emotional strength may take as much time as regaining physical strength. As you improve physically and are able to resume regular activities you should feel better. Just knowing in advance that these feelings are natural may help. Treating yourself to something special—a new outfit, a new hairdo, a walk in the woods, dinner out—can make a difference. Perhaps your most important challenge will be to think of yourself in a new way.

You! A Member
of Your Health Team

"I feel confused. I don't feel a bit good and have a lot of headaches and stomach pains. When I go to see my doctor, all he says is that I'm run down. I know that already! I lost my husband two years ago and I haven't gotten over it yet. Now I'm beginning to have trouble with my period.

"I have four kids and I feel worried about some of them. My two older kids are married and they don't have enough health insurance. One already has a baby with a lot of allergies, and that's costing them a bundle. The other one is expecting in a few weeks. She and her husband are taking that course that prepares you for natural childbirth. They're hoping to have that 'rooming in' arrangement.

"Of the two kids that still live at home, I have no problem with Susan. She works at a bakery and is saving her money to buy a car. She is very sensible and is a big help to me. But what about Jimmy? He runs around a lot with his friends and I worry about him. There's no man to talk to him about sex—and I can't do it. I thought of asking my doctor—but I just don't know.

"Trouble is, every time you turn around, it costs you. And you never seem to know how much till you go to pay. Even then, you're not sure what you paid for. Their time is worth a lot of money, but they don't seem to mind keeping you waiting. And they prescribe medicine like they own stock in some drug company. Somehow, it doesn't seem fair."

• • •

Do any of these feelings seem familiar to you? Probably so. All of us are consumers, and as such, we have a vested interest in health care services. But to many the system is confusing, fragmented, unsatisfying and costly. How did it get this way and what can be done about it?

To better understand health care and health care systems today it is worthwhile to look back thirty to forty years. Medical care has changed very rapidly with scientific and technological advances. With the changes have come dissatisfaction and conflicts between consumers and care providers.

One major change is the trend toward specialization. In 1931, only 17 percent of physicians were specialists, limiting their practices to one special body system. The family physician of the thirties and forties was usually a generalist; he cared for all the health problems of all the family members regardless of sex or age. He often had a long-term relationship with the family.

With the increase in scientific knowledge, physicians found it necessary to specialize. By 1964, 61 percent of the physicians had limited their practices to speciality areas. As specialization has increased, medical care for the individual has become fragmented. The consumer, however, doesn't specialize and is caught in a complex system.

A second major change is the development of group practices. Group practice takes one of two forms: 1) several physicians of the same specialty in an office together or 2) several physicians representing a variety of specialties in the same facility. Either type of group practice increases efficiency for physicians but may mean that the consumer has to see two or more physicians for care. In addition, many group practices are utilizing additional health personnel, such as nurse practitioners, physician's assistants, and technologists, whose roles are not clearly understood by consumers. Another change having a major impact on health care is insurance. The increase in insurance plans and increased participation of the federal government have given the consumer greater ability to pay for health care and have also led to the "overuse" of hospitals.

In addition, the focus of care is changing from medical care to health care, from curative care to preventive care. Traditionally medicine has involved the diagnosis and treatment of disease. Medical care was sought when one "got sick." As medicine has been able to eradicate many diseases that caused early death and treat others, the trend has moved toward longer life and better health.

Consumers are now looking for health care, not just medical care. They want to maintain good health, to prevent illness, to become educated in health care, and to have more of a say in matters of personal concern. The physicians provide medical care, the consumers want health care.

Because of all these changes, care providers as well as consumers are expressing discontent with today's system. The feelings of the women at the opening of this chapter would not have been prevalent several decades ago. She probably would have had a family doctor who would have given good advice about improving general mental and physical health. He would have talked with her son about sex—or she would have turned to someone else in her community. Her daughter would not have been involved in natural childbirth classes and would not be considering an alternative like "Rooming in." And her doctor would not have had the kinds of pressures which face doctors today—to provide education, to do research, and to keep abreast of a very complex body of knowledge which grows and changes at an amazing rate.

Add to this the fact that we are living in a time when human rights and human potential are very much the order of the day. No longer satisfied with mere survival, the consumer wants to be treated with dignity. The emotional climate in which medical and health care are delivered is of great concern.

And so we have a situation in which expectations are much higher because we want to assure optimal physical and mental health for each person. Together the health professional and the consumer must consider possible solutions as they work to clarify the tasks at hand and assume appropriate responsibilities to get the job done.

What are some of the things you can do?

ASSUME RESPONSIBILITY

In the preface of this book, we made the statement:

> Our bodies truly belong to us—no one else. They are
> our initial source of identity—our source of strength
> and enjoyment—our very personal responsibility.

One of the first things you can do is begin to assume that
responsibility with assertiveness. In her book *Helping Ourselves,* physician Mary C. Howell says:

> The strategies proposed, *alternatives to reliance on pro-
> fessionals for direction,* (italics ours) are simple in outline,
> although they may take years of struggle and effort to
> work into the reality of our lives. I believe that our fami-
> lies could thrive by:
>
> 1. Working to develop trusting relationships with a
> wide human network of kin, friends, neighbors, and
> others with whom we feel a sense of community;
>
> 2. Insisting that experts share with us knowledge and
> skills that we need to conduct our own affairs;
>
> 3. Utilizing the paid services of professionals at our
> own convenience—that is, only when *we* wish to do so,
> and in *our* terms.[1]

Dr. Howell continues her statement by expressing her concern for the risks we assume when we negate responsibility
for ourselves, placing our welfare in the hands of authorities
with their increasing technological capability. Her words provide us with the basis for our action.

---

[1]Mary C. Howell, *Helping Ourselves: Families and the Human
Network* (Boston: Beacon Press, 1975) See Foreward, pp. xii-xiii.

IMPROVE COMMUNICATION

Open and complete communication between health care providers and consumers is of prime importance. It is an interesting phenomenon that a consumer is willing to comparison shop, examine price tags, and ask questions when purchasing almost any goods or services from a set of dishes or a car to a hair cut or diaper service. When it comes to health care, however, consumers are reluctant to ask about services or terms of payment.

If the communication is to be effective, all members of the team—care providers and consumers—must recognize the need for this communication and work together to create the kind of atmosphere where it will be possible. This may require you, the consumer, to assume a more assertive role than you are used to—but it is your responsibility as well as your right.

Here are some of the specific things that you should become aware of and do something about.

Request information regarding procedure and policy at the doctor's office or in the hospital or clinic. When you do not feel comfortable about what is happening, say so. Remember that care providers are consumers, too, and they probably want the same considerations that you do. But no one is a mind reader, and unless thoughts and feelings are shared, communication is impossible.

Ask about the use of paraprofessionals. Find out which professional can best meet your present need. Cooperate with these providers whenever possible. It is unnecessary for a highly specialized doctor or nurse to meet your every health need.

Ask about using home care when you can. Community health services can provide homemaker aides and visiting nurses for home care services at costs far below those charged by hospitals. Again this makes the most efficient use of personnel trained in various types and at various levels of expertise.

Request a full explanation of the financial terms of your medical and health care. What will you be asked to pay and when must you pay it? What services will be offered? Are lab fees extra? Will reports be sent to you? How much do X-rays cost? Who owns the X-rays? Exactly what is included in the daily hospital rate? What costs will be extra? Do not let any question that you have about money go unanswered.

Inquire about the cost of medicine prescribed for you and members of your family. Know what you are putting into your body and why. Ask about any known side effects.

SELF-HELP

We need to keep in mind that our expectations for medical and health care are much greater than they used to be. In order for these expectations to be met, a great deal of time, energy, knowledge, and skill must be utilized. Remembering the message of Dr. Howell, we need to develop "alternatives to reliance on professionals for direction." This simply means self-reliance. In order to stay in touch with the kind and quality of health care which we receive—and to keep the costs down—the consumer can take responsibility for several things.

The efficiency and quality of your care is largely

related to how knowledgeable you are. Medical and health care providers can be very helpful in providing you with information, but you have a responsibility to inform yourself. You should know some basic principles of general health. You should be in touch with your own body. You should try to learn what you can about any health problem which you and your family may be confronting. You should seek out the information which you need to better understand the health care system. Some of the health books in the Resource section of this volume will be informative.

Groups of people can help themselves and one another. Usually these groups seek information as well as support for what may be a stressful health situation. Presently there are groups which deal with weight loss, alcoholism, child abuse, and many other health-related problems.

You will find some suggested materials in the Resource section of this book which should provide you with guidelines for forming a self-help group. Contact your community's agencies which help people find ways to meet their needs. An excellent agency is the Community Health Nursing Service. Assess the medical and health care needs and goals of your family. Are there children? How many? How old? Do you need maternity benefits? What health risks might be involved? How much insurance can you afford? For many of you, some form of health insurance may be provided as a fringe benefit where you work. Indeed, we may all be insured on a national health insurance basis relatively soon. But, for now, you must take responsibility to make some decisions about whether or not to buy health insurance or join a health maintenance plan. We have provided some suggestions for your use in the Resource section of this book.

You *can* become politicized. A number of new proposals for changing the health care system are being discussed. Two good materials to read are *The Report of the National Commission on Community Health Services* and Senator Edward Kennedy's *In Critical Condition—The Crisis In America's Health Care.* (See Resource section.) By becoming familiar with the health resources in your area, attending meetings and serving on advisory boards, and educating yourself about local and national legislation which will effect the health care system, you can direct your energies toward the kind of change you desire. Health professionals and consumers have the responsibility to work together to initiate and effect these changes.

You are a person who is continually growing and developing. In the next chapter, we will present some ideas for you to use in your exciting plans for self-development.

We are *all* consumers of health care services. Together, we are *all* responsible for working to assure the rights of each person in our human society. Individually, each person must assume the responsibility and initiative to improve communication and to develop strategies for self-help. To begin to think of yourself as an active member of your own health team is a move in the right direction.

Today

\

No woman really renounces motherhood as long as monthly or even already irregular bleedings remind her of this possibility. She feels that when a woman has ended her existence as a bearer of future life she has reached her natural end—her partial death—as a servant of the species.

(Helene Deutsch)[1]

Looking back on the anxieties which I experienced over my own hysterectomy—and continued to experience for some time—I realize that they were a result of my understanding of what it meant to be a woman. This was something I developed gradually through the years as I was growing up.

It gave me some support to learn that almost all women who were faced with a hysterectomy seemed to exper-

---

[1]Helene Deutsch, *The Psychology of Women,* Vol. II (New York: Grune and Stratton, 1945), p. 459. Reprinted by permission of Helene Deutsch.

85

ience many or all of the anxieties which I had. In a paper presented in 1971, Dr. Beverley Raphael reviewed the work of several researchers and established that most women were anxious about not being able to have more children, losing their menstrual periods, having a bad scar, growing old, dying during surgery.[2]

Using a Hysterectomy Interview Scale, Dr. Raphael discovered some interesting information about how women perceived hysterectomy as a crisis in their lives. Interactions with other people and relevant information were instrumental in their meeting the crisis successfully.

Having a hysterectomy also can greatly affect a woman's feelings of femininity. Why is this operation so emotionally loaded? Why do women have such a heavy investment in having babies, rearing children, and remaining young and beautiful forever? If we are to be able to make a healthy adjustment to this crisis in our lives, it is important that we take a look at the influences on us as we grew through infancy, girlhood, adolescence, and womanhood.

It really all starts before we are born. A question uppermost in the minds of the expectant parents and their families and friends is, "Will it be a boy or a girl?" This is the first question people ask when they are informed of a birth.

Society has expectations of how boys will behave and how girls will behave. Parents and the family serve to express those expectations to children. This is done in many ways.

---

[2]Beverley Raphael, M.B., "The Crisis of Hysterectomy," *Australian and New Zealand Journal of Psychiatry,* 6:2 (June 1972), 106-15.

Parents treat children of each gender differently, through words that are used, tone of voice, and method of physical handling.

Parents voice these expectations to their children differently: "You're a big boy, now wipe away those tears!" Or "Susie is so cute. She knows how to turn on the tears to get her way 'round Daddy!"

Parents provide models of appropriate behaviors to their growing children: "I'll put a new plug on the waffle iron. Mommy might burn the place down." (Ha ha). Or "I can't help you now. I have to sew a button on Daddy's shirt. He's all thumbs, you know." (Raised eyebrows).

During the years that a female child is growing up, her parents express the expectation to her that she will marry and have children. This is the only way to a meaningful and happy life as an adult woman. This expression is made verbally. But it is also made in other ways—providing a female child with dolls and doll furniture; driving her to dancing lessons—instead of soccer camp—because even if she doesn't become a dancer, she'll be more graceful; assuming that she, and not her brother, will be the one to baby-sit for other people or help with child care at the church or temple on the mornings they worship.

When a girl reaches menarche, the pressure to save and protect her wonderful child-producing capacity becomes intense, and the double standard is blatantly obvious. At this time the female is also bombarded with mixed messages. Mothers have been known to take their ten-year-old daughters into department stores to buy them padded bras so that they will be more popular with boys—a ridiculous exercise if you know most ten-year-old boys! Parents caution their girl children that boys like to win and don't like girls to be smarter. You have to know these things. The name of the game is to negate yourself and forget any sense of integrity in terms of your identity because the trophy—to win a male and be the mother of his children—is the ultimate social recognition.

Although parents expect that their daughter's most "natural" identity lies in the experience of motherhood and so encourage her sexuality as a means to this end, they confuse the issue by suggesting that being a good woman implies that a female must "save herself" for the man she marries. She should not want to experiment sexually with anyone else or express her sensuality in exploration with other partners. I am reminded of one of my teen-age friends who wore revealing clothes and was very suggestive in her remarks and gestures with every guy she dated. But an attempt to kiss her good-night was met with shock—"I'm not *that* kind of a girl!"

One of my college students shared with our discussion group the fact that her parents expressed very little concern about her brother when he went away to school. By the time he was a sophomore, he was living in an apartment and had a car. He was jokingly reminded by his father, "Don't do anything I wouldn't do!" However, when she started school a year later, they cautioned her endlessly about the dangers of sex and made it very clear that she could not have an apartment. They felt that girls needed the protection of dormitory living.

By the time a female reaches womanhood, her course is straight and narrow. It is narrow because her options are very limited. Trained for routine and uncreative work or no work at all, afraid to compete, reluctant to assert herself or demonstrate competency in any area other than homemaking, dependent and submissive, she waits, or searches, for a Prince Charming who will make it possible for her to live happily ever after.

As James Ramey points out, maturity is the mark of personal growth toward autonomy. An autonomous person is one who is self-contained, self-directed, and able to function without leaning on anyone else.[3] Sadly, many women do not meet this definition of maturity. But all is not lost; there is one unique, creative thing that they can do— have babies. Not only will they fulfill society's expectations, they will have human beings who will depend on them. Thus, the illusion of maturity is created.

The family, of course, is not the only institution which mediates cultural expectations to children. Schools and mass media, especially television, play a strong role in expressing and reinforcing the idea that there are very rigid roles for men and women and that a woman's role is to serve society by creating a home for a man and having his babies.

An excellent book to read on this subject is *Pronatalism: The Myth of Mom and Apple Pie.* Some two dozen selections detail and document the influence of society's institutions on gender and sexuality: curricular and extracurricular activities in schools—including books, films, teacher attitudes—community priorities, television content and process, community and religious programs, political pro-

---

[3]James Ramey, *Intimate Friendships* (Englewood Cliffs, N.J.: Prentice-Hall, Inc., 1976), p. 73.

cesses and resultant legislation. All of these factors are at work, influencing the kind of people we become.[4]

But you don't have to read a book to learn this. If you simply examine your daily life, you can see these forces at work. A book was mailed to me by a publisher recently. It is a textbook to be considered for a course on the family for young people. Although it contains chapters which discuss birth control and the problem of world population, the author makes this statement at the opening of *his* chapter on the birth of the first child:

> The birth of the first child is a high point in marriage. It expresses in visible new life the strength and vitality of the invisible bond of love between husband and wife. Especially for the woman, the coming of a child has great significance. It is a confirmation of her womanhood, a fulfillment of the unique role she alone can perform.[5]

This book was published in 1974. There are wonderfully mature human beings with active, exciting, childless marriages who would take issue with the idea that their bond of love is invisible. And how terrible to state that the coming of the first child has special significance for the *woman*!

The amount of time that women spend discussing pregnancy, having babies, caring for them as they grow up, shopping for and preparing food, and keeping houses and

---

[4]Ellen Peck and Judith Senderowitz, *Pronatalism: The Myth of Mom and Apple Pie* (New York: Thomas Y. Crowell Co., 1975).

[5]Edith L. Potter, "Pregnancy," *Successful Marriage* by Fishbein/Fishbein, is paraphrased in Robert K. Kelley, *Courtship, Marriage, and the Family,* second ed. (New York: Harcourt, Brace, Jovanovich, 1974), p. 473. Reprinted by permission of Harcourt, Brace, Jovanovich, Inc.

clothes immaculately clean is astounding. But it becomes frightening when you realize that this is also happening on television. A study made a few years ago established that the average five-year-old child spends approximately fifty-five hours a week watching television. More recent figures state that the average child spends more time watching television over her/his lifetime than going to school!

And then there is the board game, *LIFE*. Players drive around the board in a small plastic car. Blue tokens are used for make, pink for females. Males remain in the driver's seat throughout the game. Females move over to the passenger side when (hopefully!) they get married. And, of course, there are bonuses for having babies!

My own fears and anxieties seemed to center around four main concerns: sexual, physical dependency, damage to my body, and death. Although some of these concerns are related to any kind of surgery, all of them were related, for me, to my identity as a woman.

I did not want to lose my capacity to bear children. Regular menstrual periods signaled to me that all was well on that front, and so, understandably, I did not want those periods to cease. I wanted to remain sexually active and sexually attractive.

I have always been an active person and, more recently, quite autonomous. I was worried about that period of time when I would need others to do things for me. After all, I was the nuturing figure who provided care for everyone else. Would I be less of a woman if I had to be cared for by others in my family?

My body had to be as perfect as I could make it. A woman knows this. Would the scar be obvious and ugly? Would it show when I wore hip-hugger shorts? How much would my skin tone and body tone deteriorate with a sudden loss of estrogen? How fast would my hair turn grey? How fat would I get—how soon?

Death speaks for itself. Surgery is a risk. Not only did I not want to die, but as the mother of five children, I had to live!

It is very obvious that women are programmed to have a strong identity with their reproductive systems. Certainly society needs to replenish itself with a limited number of children, and quality nurturing and protection must be provided for these children.

But I now realize that many of my concerns were in my belief that the very core of my being would be weakened or taken away when I had my hysterectomy. I know that many, many women share these feelings. This is a result of our being socialized to focus our identities on the capacity to reproduce. However, research reported in the May and July 1977 issues of *Human Behavior* newsmagazine (Eschen and Huyck, 1976, and Meikle, Brody, and Pysh, 1977) provides clear evidence that the women who were studied had a more positive attitude about hysterectomy after they had this surgery than did women who had not undergone hysterectomy. And the fact of hysterectomy did not cause any greater emotional problem than comparable organ surgery. Next in this book we discuss some of the specifics in terms of helping ourselves and our children define ourselves in ways which are not as limiting as this.

Kiss Cinderella
Goodbye

The story line is familiar. A young girl is hopelessly trapped. Her adversary is a wicked stepmother or evil godmother. The only thing that can save her from her lot in life is to have Prince Charming enter center stage and take her as his bride to a better life—a life in which, it is promised, she will live happily ever after. The story could be *Cinderella*—or *Sleeping Beauty* or *Snow White.* The elements are all the same. Implicit in these stories is the message that females cannot take responsibility for themselves. Submissiveness is presented as an innate female trait. The only way a girl can become a true adult female and find a way out of her present situation is to leave on the strong arm of Prince Charming.

She will, of course, take her submissive personality with her. And therein lies the greater trap! A human being who is subordinate and dependent cannot be autonomous and responsible. It is difficult to imagine living happily ever after under those circumstances.

If these stories were only fairy tales, there would not be as great a cause for concern. But the basic story line, with a few variations, is all around us in contemporary society. In this chapter, specific suggestions will be presented—suggestions of ways in which we might sift these implications out of our daily lives and build a healthier climate for the psychosexual and psychosocial development of our children and youth. If we can increase their opportunities for development into self-actualizing adults, we can increase the possibility that they will want to assume responsibility for themselves rather than wait passively for someone else to make critical life decisions for them.

The first awareness that a baby has of herself as a separate being is an awareness of her body. This awareness is developed through many sensorimotor experiences including stretching, sucking her thumb and other objects, studying her fingers and toes, touching and feeling everything in her grasp—her own body included. As she grows older, she begins to define herself in other ways. Many of the impressions she gains about herself are learned as she relates to other people and figures out what they expect of her. Many of these expectations are fixed by gender. Many of them are emotionally loaded in terms of the female body.

The female child who grows through girlhood and adolescence into womanhood feeling good about her body, feeling secure and confident about herself as a learner, and feeling free about her personhood, will be an autonomous adult who chooses to assume responsibility for herself and others and who is able to accept their caring for her. She will be a more competent worker, a more competent citizen, a more competent friend—and a more competent mate and parent, should she choose either of these roles. Surely, she will seek the growing paths in life.

This must be viewed as an asset in all aspects of her life. It is certainly an asset in terms of her ability to participate effectively in her own health care. She will seek until she finds a doctor she trusts; she will gain the knowledge she needs; she will cooperate in making decisions which benefit her; she will question or reject those which she thinks will not.

Now, let's examine some of the things which we can do to facilitate the development of children into more competent and responsible adults. Let's look at ways we can increase awareness of ourselves and the roles we model. Let's examine our expectations of children and the ways in which we communicate these expectations. Let's consider how we can attend to their environment, effecting change where we can and helping children to develop the ability to select those experiences and materials designed to help them be free.

There is a saying that goes something like this—"I cannot hear what you are saying because what you are doing is making so much noise." The spoken expectations of adults are often in conflict with their actions. Because adults who are parenting, teaching, or otherwise relating to children and youth serve as models for those young people, the first suggestion is that adults become aware of themselves as people.

There are several ways in which this might be done.

For some people, just thinking about it honestly might be enough. But for most people, it is more effective to work with someone else or with a group of people. It is good to have goals in mind, such as trying to determine one's values and priorities. Another goal might be to determine attitudes about certain people or issues and see if these change as levels of consciousness are raised.

One way to determine our attitudes about other people is to put ourselves into situations in which we experience what it must be like to be someone else. We could modify the experiment which a classroom teacher tried with her group. Those people with blue eyes were required to sit in the back of the room and were ostracized by the rest of the group. After awhile, they had a better understanding of how people feel when they are stereotyped and mistreated on the basis of a physical characteristic.

One homemaker's attitudes about the exciting career world of men changed when she became the major breadwinner in her family. With her consciousness at a new level, she became more sensitive to the pressures on men and the many personal compromises they have to make.

Reading—alone or with others—is a useful way to increase awareness of self, of others, of values and attitudes. Several books which should be helpful are listed under Resources.

Joining a group of friends in forming a people's group has been effective for some adults. There may be an existing structure for such groups in a nearby community center, church, or college. One friend was delighted when the large corporation for whom her husband works designed some personal growth sessions for their employees. Her husband now has a new approach to their baby daughter.

An important part of this self-assessment is to look at the roles we assume and how we play them. Men are "telling" children something when they do not cry, will not admit to mistakes, cannot sew on a button. Women are "telling" children something when they do not assert themselves, will not make decisions, cannot change a tire. We are "telling" children that it is unacceptable to express feelings, to develop behaviors naturally, or to learn the skills and knowledge which every competent person should have.

Keep in mind that it isn't enough to tell a child that we expect her to grow up and manage her financial affairs competently. Mothers and teachers must model this behavior. The adult female who moans, "I'm so helpless when it comes to money—I can never balance my checkbook," is delivering her message loud and clear!

Because they are young and look to us for what is right and wrong, because they want so much to please and be accepted, children are vulnerable. They will behave in the ways we want them to behave—or at least they will *try*. They will do this, even if it means denying themselves. And so it becomes critical to examine our "wants"—the expectations we have for children.

Most people would probably agree that they want children to grow up to be responsible, to get a good education, to be able to think, solve problems, and make decisions. But isn't it too easy to stop there? What do we mean by these words—and do we mean the same things for females as we do for males?

What *is* a good education? One answer is that a good education fosters the gaining of those knowledges and skills which are necessary for a person to function optimally. Lillian Smith[1] has written:

> The whole world is a man's home and there should be no place in it where he is not welcome. The whole world is in a man's heart, also, and there should be no place in it where he fears to enter.

Substituting the word person, we can say that a woman needs to be at home in the world and with herself. This is possible only to the extent that she is knowledgeable about that world and herself and is skillful in applying that knowledge.

All children need to learn practical skills as they are growing up. All children need to learn how to have fun. All children need to learn how to do something that will earn them a living. All children need to learn how to think, to solve problems, to make decisions.

Our expectations for them must not be limited by stereotypes but should be tempered by knowledge of them as individuals. One person, male or female, may have good manual dexterity and may enjoy working on things with small parts. Another person may have some physiologically based limitation for this kind of work or may simply be too impatient. Individual potentials, needs, and interests must always be considered.

---

[1] Writer Lillian Smith was devoted to the cause of racial integration and equality for all human beings.

With this in mind, we should expect many female children to be capable of understanding electricity and learning how to make electrical repairs. Many female children can develop into competent athletes and participate successfully in both team and individual sports. Female children can be educated to earn a living. Female children can learn to solve problems, to be decisive, to be direct. In short, female children can learn to be responsible for themselves. As we stated earlier, one of the most significant ways we communicate our expectations to children is to model appropriate behaviors ourselves. When children see that we are free, they will know that this is a good thing to be. And they will be comfortable with the idea that it's OK to be what you want to be.

It is important that our verbal communication with children be open, direct, and very clear. We should share, appropriately, what we think and feel about our expectations. We should focus on the behavior, not on the worth, of the child as a person. For example, it is honest to say, "I don't like to be kicked, and I can't allow you to do that." But it would be destructive to say, "You are a bad girl for kicking me." Help her to think through what is right for her and to take the responsibility for her developing self. Several good books about adult-child relations are available. Although the suggested methods of communications differ in some ways, most of them share the same basic belief: children are people capable of learning to deal with reasonable adult expectations and of working out an identity for themselves in a supportive emotional climate. Some of these books are listed in the Resources section of this volume. Another way that we communicate our expectations to children is in the way that we do, or do not, arrange and prepare their environment and help them to learn to examine that environment critically, selecting and adding the experiences which will help them to be free. Painted in huge white letters on the red brick wall which helps to protect a day care play-yard in the Boston area are the words

POWER TO YOUNG PEOPLE

Stop and think about the significance of those words. Each suppressed group, in turn, has met and marched and demanded their rights to a proud identity. Each group was able to gain effective control by demonstrating their economic and political power.

But children don't have money to spend and they cannot vote. No political leader of stature has ever campaigned under the banner

KIDS ARE A PRIORITY!

In his book *Escape From Childhood,*[2] John Holt helps us to examine our attitudes about children . . . attitudes that cause us to deal with children in ways that are "sentimental" and "cute." The end result is that we deny children the respect they deserve as they go about the exciting and serious task of growing up to become responsible and growing adults.

We tend to pat children on their heads, swoop them off their feet and carry them around, speak to them in patronizing tones, and ask them questions with hidden agendas. As we observe ourselves and others, it becomes

---

[2]John Holt, *Escape From Childhood* (New York: Ballantine Books Inc., 1976).

obvious that we very often invade the rights of childen by satisfying our adult needs to touch and fondle, or feel superior, regardless of the child's wishes. One of the very first things we can do is search for evidences of chauvinism. Think about the language we use, the things we pay attention to and the things we ignore, the pictures we use, the ways in which homes and classrooms are set up, the kinds of activities we foster and those we ignore or refuse altogether. Examine the books we read or give to children and the recordings we make available for their use. Listen to some of the messages they hear over the radio. Take a hard look at the content of television programs and commercials, newspaper and magazine advertisements, and motion pictures. We find, of course, that crippling sex role stereotypes abound!

Is there anything we can do about this in a world so widely invaded by the technology of the news media? Yes —there are two important things we can do!

First, we can have an impact on the child's environment. We can replace negative influences with positive materials and experiences.

> Remove "cute" pictures from the home and classroom— pictures which depict girls as dewyeyed little darlings, cuddling equally dewy-eyed little kittens, and boys as impish little ragamuffins, breaking windows in their athletic misadventures. Replace them with photographs and paintings which present human beings with integrity. Recently, several popular magazines ran ads which depicted children and elders from several ethnic groups in full-page color photographs. An inexpensive set of four photographs of men in the nurturing role is available. (See Resources.)

Remove books and records which stereotyped people. Replace them with materials that affirm individuality. These can be purchased or borrowed from your library. The Resources section lists sources which can be used to develop criteria for evaluating materials. A selected group of children's books is included.

Arrange your home and classroom so that both male and female children have access to space, equipment, and materials which will enable them to develop skills in activities which appeal to them. Encourage all children to try a variety of activities. For example, blocks and trucks should not be confined to a boy's room—or homemaking equipment to a girl's room. Art activities should sometimes include the use of a saw, hammer, and materials such as wood, metal pieces, nails, and other hardware.

Remember to comment on the handsome sweater that a boy is wearing and on how well a girl climbs. We all enjoy the feeling of positive reinforcement.

Work in your community to ensure equal opportunity for males and females in recreational and educational programs, and evaluate materials available at your library.

Participate in the activities of such groups as Action for Children's Television and use your economic and political power to remove sexism, racism, and violence from television programs and commercials.

Secondly, we can help children to develop the skills needed to evaluate materials and experiences which are available to them and to reject those which will limit them. This is the more difficult action to take because it means we must spend the time necessary to help them develop their values and learn to evaluate and make decisions. Then, we must direct some of our energy into supporting them as they implement those decisions.

It isn't easy for a boy who chooses not to fight back. The girl who is direct and assertive isn't being ladylike. The boy who wants to study dance is suspect. The girl who confronts a teacher over the drudgery of a classroom is not accepted.

Supporting children through the process of evaluating their experiences and making choices is an important endeavor and one on which the home and school should work together. The school offers a peer group setting. Peer group acceptance and understanding are very important to children as they learn to act independently and assume responsibility for those actions.

A mother buys her young adolescent daughter a padded bra. A teacher encourages his female students in the womanly art of flirting. A radio announcer softly murmurs, "Since the day he slipped that ring on her finger, her days have been filled with sunshine." A toy manufacturer designs a Sunshine Family—"complete" with mother, father, and a child named "Sweets." A TV writer creates a commercial in which two women become ecstatic over a detergent which will make baby's diapers whiter and softer. And women everywhere are encouraged to take Geritol so "he" will keep them.

Fiction! *No!* Facts. The world of Cinderella is still very much with us. And until adults make the decision to take action—to kiss Cinderella goodbye—little girls will keep growing up with the goal of finding a man to take care of them and provide them with that happy-ever-after life. And little boys will keep growing up with the burden of trying to do just that.

Today
Is the First Day . . .

In all our lives there are choices to be made; it is up to us to make those choices for ourselves.

For some, making thoughtful decisions and acting with commitment is already an established pattern. For others, there is a need to take greater initiative, even to find new directions. For many, the idea of assuming responsibility for self, of making daily as well as life decisions, offers quite a new option. But all of us find life more satisfying and fulfilling as we take hold of this idea and begin to assume responsibility for self-development.

It will be helpful to review some of the understandings we have about ourselves. Erik Erikson has described eight stages of psychosocial development. Others have contributed to our knowledge as well. Some suggested readings are provided in the Resource section. Erikson focuses on the ego development of the human being. Each of us is faced with working out the problems of each stage through a process of "social interaction" in which we interact with ourselves and others. This process is lifelong because we never stop growing and developing. Although it is possible to move through a stage without resolving the crisis, the growing person tries to meet the challenge of each stage with a positive attitude. The psychosocial stages are:

Trust vs. Mistrust (ages birth to 2 years) in which the infant establishes herself as a worthwhile person in relationship with her nurturing figures.

Autonomy vs. Doubt (ages 2 and 3 years) in which the child views herself as a person who has some control.

Initiative vs. Guilt (ages 4 and 5 years) in which the child learns to initiate activities and projects. Some of this takes the form of asking questions. Much of the ability to participate in this stage and the previous stage is dependent upon the child's competency in motor skills and language.

Industry vs. Inferiority (ages 6 to 12) in which the child establishes herself as a competent person, able to accomplish what she starts out to do.

Identity vs. Role Confusion (ages 12 to 18) in which the adolescent tries to sort out the many definitions of herself and synthesize them into a definition of herself as a person with an identity which is acceptable.

Intimacy vs. Isolation (young adulthood) in which the task is to maintain the identity of the previous stage while developing the ability to be close to another person—to care about that person and share intimately. These are friendships which may, but need not, include sexuality. For many, it is a period for establishing a family.

Generativity vs. Self-Absorption (middle age) in which the person not only develops concerns about persons in her intimate circle of family and friends, but learns to care about future generations and the kind of world in which they will live. Everyone who works through this stage successfully will direct a great deal of energy toward trying to improve the world for now and the future.

Integrity vs. Despair (old age) in which the effectiveness of our lives up to this point is reflected. Whether or not we can look back on our lives and feel good about the way we have lived them is critical at this point. To find satisfaction and pleasure in our old age is important to each of us. Without this sense of integrity, we despair.

The realistic person knows that the tasks inherent in each of these stages are apt to reappear in life and will require more work.

As adults, we experience the last three of these psychosocial tasks: intimacy, generativity, and integrity. Working through these requires that we use initiative, make some choices, and act with commitment. It is important that we begin to assume responsibility for our own development NOW.

It is also helpful—in trying to understand ourselves —to consider the social conditions which are unique to our period of human history. The technology which pervades and invades every aspect of our lives today brings with it both positive and negative dimensions.

We have learned more about ourselves. This is good. But we are now faced with greater demands to grow and improve ourselves than ever before. We have a much improved standard of living in terms of health care, travel, communication, and opportunities for education and recreation, but we often do not have the time to take advantage of these opportunities. In addition, we are plagued with diseases which are a result of improper diet, insufficient exercise, dependence on stimulants and depressants, and our inability to cope with a tense and stress-filled society.

In his book *The Relaxation Response,* [1] Dr. Herbert Benson points out that physically and psychologically threatening and stressful situations abound in our modern world. The response to these situations by fighting or fleeing is elicited very, very often. Most of the time we neither fight nor flee. Our bodies are forced to "live with" unrelieved tension. Benson suggests that we learn to elicit a relaxation response in order to cope with stress.

It is encouraging to listen to Dr. Benson and to read other material which emphasizes our ability to act on behalf of ourselves. People like Carl Rogers and Abraham Maslow help us to understand that we have the potential to work through the challenges of life. We have the creative potential to be self-actualizing.

A friend has said that each of us must experience a personal revolution. Something has to happen inside of us. We have to *want* to do something, to be *ready* to make a commitment, before we can make any meaningful changes in our lives. A network of resources is available to us; support is there. We must want to use these resources and this support.

In the two preceding chapters, we developed some suggestions of actions that will make a difference for yourself and for other people. In this chapter, we want to focus

---

[1] Herbert Benson, *The Relaxation Response* (New York: William Morrow and Co., Inc., 1975).

on you. What are some of the things which you can do today to take care of your personal needs as a self-actualizing adult?

Consider a statement made about a decade ago at an early childhood meeting in the first days of the movement to raise the consciousness of the world. It describes the way many of us were raised.

> When you watch young children at school, you see little girls practicing diligently in their workbooks, learning to read and print earlier than little boys do. As you look around the room, you can see their gold-star papers lining the walls and filling the bulletin boards—announcing that they have mastered the skills of tying their shoelaces, or counting to one hundred, or knowing their number facts. Little girls almost always hand in more book reports than little boys do.
>
> You see little boys building with blocks and making up games with their own rules. You see little boys exploring and investigating, taking things apart and asking question after question. Much of their resistance to the grind of academic expectations is dismissed with a whimsical shrug of tolerant shoulders—"Boys will be boys, you know."
>
> And when these young children grow up, the little boys become men who direct large companies, design and build bridges, and create magnificent paintings, sculptures, music, and literature. And the little girls? They become women who stay home and have the babies of these men—and iron their shirts.[2]

We may not be ironing shirts anymore and we seem to be having fewer babies, but are we developing the creative

---

[2]Corrine Maddocks, Goddard College, Plainfield, Ohio.

potential that is ours? Having babies and making a home constitutes an important task—and one which can be enhanced by a creative approach to the job. But for many women, the task is limiting. They find that they need something more. Many women do not have children; they are not "programmed" into childrearing during their early adult years. The challenge of developing creative potential is just as real for them.

Madeline Gray, in her book *The Changing Years,*[3] has a wonderful chapter entitled, "Not *The* Change but *Another* Change." She suggests you practice right now saying "another change," or "the changing years." For as you move into the years of generativity, you are moving into the years of maximum influence. Generativity not only involves a feeling of obligation to care for others but also a commitment to self-development—to fulfilling one's own creative potential.

In considering the development of this creative potential, let's look at four areas which can profit if you approach them with a positive attitude: work, avocational interests, friendships, and health.

WORK

Every human being thrives on finding meaningful, productive work to do. This work can be done on a volunteer basis as well as for a wage or salary. The training for

---

[3]Madeline Gray, *The Changing Years* (New York: New American Library, 1973).

this work and its early implementation usually occur during the periods of "identity" and "intimacy"—those years we call adolescence and young adulthood. Some people actually do make a thoughtful choice and receive the training they need to begin their life work.

Many other people, however, do not work this task out to their satisfaction. You may be one of these people. Perhaps you interrupted school to start a family or to help your parents with problems they may have had. Perhaps you chose work you really do not want to do. Perhaps, as you have grown into middle age, new interests have opened up which you would like to explore in terms of a career.

You *can do* something about this! We aren't suggesting that it is an easy thing to do. You are not alone. Many women are "back in school," working toward high school diplomas, receiving vocational training, or studying toward a bachelor or graduate degree.

You will have to take the initiative to contact your local or state Board of Education, Employment Security Office, or Human or Social Services Agency. Depending upon your financial situation, there may be federally funded programs which will train you for a new career. Financial aid, in the form of grants, loans, work-study, or assistantships, is available. There are a growing number of nontraditional education and training programs which make it possible for you to study without prolonged absences from your home base or present job.

Why not start by going to your local high school and asking to speak with a guidance counselor? He or she may not be able to give you the specific help you need but could direct you to the most appropriate place for you to begin on this very important task of finding meaningful work for yourself.

AVOCATIONAL INTERESTS

As we think about this area of our lives, it is interesting to consider how vital it is to our older years—the years of "integrity." However, we direct so much of our time and energy in the earlier periods of our lives toward achieving status, earning money, and raising a family that we often neglect to develop other interests.

Whatever your age is now, it is important for you to take stock of this very important aspect of your development. Are there forms of exercise which you enjoy on a regular basis? Do some of these get you outdoors? Are you in some kind of consistent touch with the arts—either through singing or dancing or painting *or* through attending concerts, museums, movies, or plays? Do you read regularly, for pleasure as well as for information? Are there things which you enjoy doing with your hands?

Most communities have cultural, recreational, and educational programs free of charge—or available at a nominal charge. Sometimes these are available at your high school or through a community college or recreation program.

If what you want isn't available, why wouldn't it be possible to get together with a group of people who would like to learn to fix cars, or make furniture, or square dance, and find someone who would work with the group for the satisfaction of helping? A self-help group is not an unreasonable expectation. Everyone has something to teach! *Someone* has to help get things going.

FRIENDSHIPS

In his timely and supportive book *Intimate Friendships,* James Ramey helps us to realize that we limit ourselves when we become locked into the possessive relationships which many of us have grown up to think we need.

Our friendships are very often narrowly defined. We are raised with the maxim that we are judged by the people with whom we keep company. These people must be of a certain social status, age level, political opinion, or religious or ethnic group. And these people most certainly should not pose a sexual threat to our other relationships.

This narrow definition tends to build a wall around our social selves. But we can do something to tear that wall down, brick by brick. We can work hard to strengthen the friendships we already have. And we can risk the reaching out to make new friends.

Taking that risk is not an easy thing to do. It means we must believe in our intrinsic worth as people and learn to trust and be trusted. In recognizing that other people need us as much as we need them, we lay a very good foundation for finding and developing new friendships. A very important beginning in this commitment is to learn to care for ourselves.

PHYSICAL AND MENTAL HEALTH

One's appearance depends on many things, personality, grooming, health, and mental outlook, to name a few. Today's society is so geared to youth and looking young that many women feel that having a hysterectomy or entering menopause spells doom; the end of reproductive function means the start of old age. However, most women have at least a third of their lives ahead of them at this time!

You will age with or without the ovaries present, but it need not be abrupt or threatening. Proper attention to diet, rest, exercise, grooming, and general physical and mental health will keep you just as feminine and attractive as you have always been.

Good physical and mental health encompass many things. Regular medical checkups are of extreme importance whether you are approaching menopause or past it; whether you have had a hysterectomy or not. During the middle years, the entire body undergoes many changes. Attention to these changes helps to assure good health.

For example:

Eye changes occur when the lens becomes firmer and less resilient, interfering with accommodation. These changes may occur gradually, subtly. You might not be aware of them without an eye examination.

Dental care takes on increasing importance. Gum disease is more common in middle age, and teeth may loosen. Proper care can ward off infection and, perhaps, even a need for dentures.

Heart disease, cancer, and stroke are still the leading causes of death. The incidence of all three increases after the age of 40. Physical examinations can pick up early signs and symptoms, and early treatment could add years to your life.

So the first thing you can do is see that you receive regular medical and dental care.

Then take some of the more common middle-age concerns in turn and see what you can do about them.

Skin Changes

Skin changes have nothing to do with whether you have a uterus or not. They occur as fat pads beneath the skin are absorbed and elasticity diminishes. Wrinkling often occurs in the face and neck and in the breast. There may be a loss of tone, and tiny blood vessels may appear at the surface of the skin. As these changes occur, your best move is to change cosmetics. Remember, heavy makeup accentuates rather than conceals and the use of lighter, flatter tones and less makeup will improve your appearance. Lubrication with creams and lotions will prevent a dry skin look. Facial exercises help keep the skin firm. They are easily learned and can be done anytime. (See Resource section.)

The skin on the hands and other parts of the body may also feel dry and itchy. It, too, can be kept moist with creams and lotions.

A word about cosmetic hormone creams. Recently, a number of cosmetic manufacturers have put out creams containing estrogen that "will make you young and glamorous." Studies done by a dermatologist in New York proved otherwise: the creams contained very little hormone, and most of it was lost in rubbing, very little was absorbed. Added to the fact that they cost about five times as much as other creams, there is very little to recommend them.

Breast Changes

The breasts may also lose tone and appear wrinkled or feel "flabby." If so, a well-fitted, supportive bra will eliminate any sagging. Beyond this, the single most important thing any woman can do for herself is to examine her breasts regularly. Breast changes are almost always discovered by women themselves, and early detection is one of the best preventions of cancer. The American Cancer Society has two excellent leaflets on how to examine your breasts, and Dr. Davis describes the method in his book. Make this a regular practice!

Weight Gain

The loss of skin elasticity is no reason to gain weight. There may be a tendency to put on weight in the forties and fifties, but this has nothing to do with hysterectomy.

It occurs when you eat more and exercise less. "Middle-age spread" cannot be blamed on surgery or menopause. It is easy to get careless with eating habits, to snack between meals, to nibble at coffee klatches or club meetings. Once children are grown and no longer at home, there may be less "running around" and less exercise to burn up the extra calories. Continued vigilance over the amount and type of food you eat and sufficient exercise prevent excessive weight gain.

The best place to begin is to keep track of exactly what you eat for a week. Be honest—list everything. Then take a look at the list and see where the extra calories are coming from, where you could cut down or substitute a low calorie snack.

Learn the approximate caloric values of food you ordinarily eat. For example, chocolate ice cream contains twice as many calories as vanilla; oranges contain twice as many as grapefruit. You can still enjoy ice cream and citrus fruit and yet cut calories in half with alternate choices.

A well-balanced diet is essential to health regardless of caloric intake. Daily menus should include the basic four food groups: the milk group consisting of milk and milk products; the meat group consisting of meat, fish, poultry, and eggs; the vegetable and fruit group; and the bread and cereal group.

Developing new dietary habits takes time. Because people eat for a wide variety of reasons other than hunger, new practices may involve far more than simple menu changes. But if you are patient—and determined—you can help keep weight from becoming a problem for you.

Note: Rapid weight reduction can be hazardous. Fad diets can be dangerous. If you are excessively overweight, or in doubt about diet, be sure to consult your doctor.

Exercise

Earlier we asked, "Are there forms of exercise which you enjoy on a regular basis?" Exercise is the answer to increasing muscle tone and distributing weight. This does not mean marathon sessions at a gym or costly formal programs. Continue with the sports you enjoy. If you don't enjoy sports, begin with a few simple exercises and gradually build them up. Many community organizations have exercise or yoga groups, as do some television stations.

Exercise improves circulation to nearly all parts of the body. As the years go by, the speed with which you do an activity may be reduced, but not skill or accuracy. Exercise should be regular—not in sudden spurts. Lungs need oxygen and your heart needs circulation—slack muscles cannot meet these demands. Fresh air activities such as walking, bike riding, golf, tennis, and the like help the muscles to increase in tone and in function. The more you use—the less you lose!

The human body thrives with activity, adapts to meet increased demands, and ultimately works more efficiently. Physical limitations are individual, so your exercise program must be tailored to your needs and abilities. You are competing only with yourself—to make the most of *your* potential. As the Council on Aging tells you—"Get off your rocker and get going!"

Sexual Function

One of the fears most often expressed is that hysterectomy and/or oophorectomy will seriously damage sexual activity. There is no relationship between enjoyment of sexual intercourse and the presence of reproductive organs. Sexual desire and desirability do not disappear. Femininity does not disappear. Attitudes play the biggest part in healthy sexual relationships. In fact, many women express a new freedom in sexual expression when the fear of pregnancy is gone. The studies of Masters and Johnson have shown that despite physical changes that occur with menopause, the response of the clitoris and the ability of the vagina to accept an erect penis does not change.[4] Some women actually experience a heightened sex drive. As children are grown and leave home, they describe this period of life as "a second honeymoon."

Problems that arise in the middle years may be due to tension from overwork, financial worries, or simply from worry and fear that sexual function will change. Men are especially prone to concerns at this time. Much of their self-esteem is tied to their ability to perform sexually. As they approach their fifties, their ability may be tapering off. They worry too. Menopause is not a time when you give less—it is a time to give more.

Masters and Johnson, in *The Pleasure Bond,*[5] stress the importance of communicating, of keeping in touch, of making the effort to reach out to your partner . . . and making a commitment. This is the cement that binds people together.

They state that if a man and a woman are committed to the enjoyment of their own sexual natures and to each other as sexual persons, and are willing to experiment with new techniques, middle-age sexuality can be most satisfying.

The important things to remember are your needs and desires for sexual expression and that your abilities to

[4]William Masters and Virginia Johnson, *Human Sexual Response* (Boston: Little, Brown and Company, 1966).

[5]William Masters and Virginia Johnson, *The Pleasure Bond* (Boston: Little, Brown and Company, 1974).

maintain sexual performance and response need not change after hysterectomy. If problems arise, discuss them with your doctor to determine possible causes and solutions.

Emotions

Emotional outlook is important. In spite of what you may have heard, most women experience few, if any, major problems during menopause or following a hysterectomy. All women do experience changes and adjustments throughout their lives—from puberty to pregnancy to menopause. Feelings of nervousness, irritability, and depression normally come and go.

It is the "idle" woman who experiences the greatest emotional problems. The woman who is "on the go" in a job, who participates in community activities, and who is involved in creative endeavors will be busy and feel useful and needed. Many women acquire new skills and develop new interests during these years of generativity. They become more vibrant and more interesting.

The women who succumb to abnormal depression during this time do so because of special individual situations and stresses which were already present. Their experience is coincidental to, not because of, menopause. Dr. William Menninger states that the best therapy for depression is love: learn to love yourself, other people, work, and play. Start thinking of yourself with kindness. Respect yourself for the good person you are. Learn new things and develop new attitudes. Remember that it is far better to do something you may feel is useless or even silly, than to do nothing at all. As long as you are busy and involved, you will be emotionally safe and sound.

Each of you will move through life's stages; some will move more easily than others. You have the capacity to make choices for yourself. In today's society, you will find more support for those choices than ever before.

Whatever you can do, or dream you can, begin it.
Boldness has genius, power and magic in it.

GOETHE

Resources

This section contains selected and categorized resources to help you know where to turn to find ways to help yourself. Each "turning" will lead to new resources—new books, new people, new ideas. We hope you find it of help.

PEOPLE

Many of the people who can best help you are right in your own community. Look in your telephone directory for a Women's Health Center. The title may begin with the name of your community, county, or state.

It is also wise to explore community resources through your municipal office, Chamber of Commerce, newspapers, hospitals, nursing associations, schools, or churches.

Excellent source books for locating organized groups are *The New Woman's Survival Catalog* and *The New Woman's Survival Source Book*. Both of these are detailed in the following section of *Resources*. Four feminist retreats suggested in the latter (p. 241) are:

A Woman's Place
Athol, N.Y. 02810
518-623-9541

Emma's Place
P.O. Box 717
Grover City, Calif. 93433
805-489-9633

Femø
75 Kontor
Kvindehuset
Abenra 26
DK-1124 Copenhagen K.
Denmark

Womanshare
1531 Grays Creek Rd.
Grants Pass, Ore. 97526

Two action groups you might want to join (also listed in *Source Book,* p. 34) are: The Women's Caucus of the American Public Health Association (Jayne Graves, Chairperson), 444½ Curson Ave., Los Angeles, Ca., and the National Women's Health Lobby, with sponsors in several cities.

Other groups of people who are organized to help you are listed here. Write to them and ask to be included on their mailing lists. You will then be kept informed of materials they are developing or programs they plan to offer. This will help you begin to develop your own network of resources.

Adult Education Association
1225 Nineteenth Street
Washington, D.C. 20036

**The Citizen's Advisory Council
on the Status of Women**
Dept. of Labor Building
Room 1336
Washington, D.C. 20210

Community Health Services
(Look in phone book under
Visiting Nurses Assoc. and
Public Health Department.)

**Joint Commission on
Accreditation of Hospitals**
645 North Michigan Avenue
Chicago, Illinois 60611
(For accredited hospitals
in your area)

**Sex Information and
Education Council (SIECUS)**
1855 Broadway
New York, N.Y. 10023

Women in Midstream
University of Washington YWCA
4224 University Way, N.E.
Seattle, Washington 98105
206-632-4747
(Women studying and distributing
information related to menopause, estrogen, etc.)

American Cancer Society
219 East 42nd Street
New York, N.Y. 10017

Common-Unity[1]
Another Place Farm
Rd. 103
Greenville, N.H. 03048
603-878-1510

Group Health Assoc. of America
1321 Fourteenth Street, N.W.
Washington, D.C. 20005
(For comprehensive medical
care plans)

Planned Parenthood
515 Madison Avenue
New York, N.Y. 10022

Public Citizen
P.O. Box 19404
Washington, D.C. 20036
(Includes a citizen's group
in "Health Research")

Lollipop Power, Inc.
P.O. Box 1171
Chapel Hill, N.C. 27514
(People working to free
children of sex role stereotypes)

U.S. Public Health Service
U.S. Government Printing Office
Washington, D.C.

---

[1]This is a New England-based group interested in self-help
in all aspects of our lives, including health. They hold healing fairs, are
interested in alternate methods of healing, and are part of a network of
resources. They publish a newsletter.

READING MATERIALS

This is a selected list of material. We have tried to choose books, pamphlets, and articles which you can find in local libraries and stores. In some instances, we have provided addresses so that you may order items of interest to you.

If you have access to past copies of popular magazines, you might like to review a *Reader's Guide to Periodical Literature* in order to locate several articles on hysterectomy which have been printed during the last eight years.

• • •

Women's Sourcebooks

COWAN, BELITA, *Women's Health Care: Resources, Writings, Bibliographies.*
Available from:
Belita Cowan
556 Second Street
Ann Arbor, Michigan 48103

RENNIE, SUSAN, AND KIRSTEN GRIMSTEAD, eds., *The New Woman's Survival Catalog.* New York: Coward, McCann, and Geoghegan, 1973; New York: Berkeley Publishing Corporation, 1973.

RENNIE, SUSAN, AND KIRSTEN GRIMSTEAD, eds., *The New Woman's Survival Sourcebook.* New York: Alfred A. Knopf, 1975.

Self-Health

GENERAL

BOSTON WOMEN'S HEALTH COLLECTIVE, *Our Bodies, Ourselves* (revised and expanded). New York: Simon and Schuster, 1972.

RUSH, ANNE KENT, *Getting Clear.* New York: Random House: The Bookworks, 1973.

> Random House: The Bookworks
> 1409 Fifth Avenue
> Berkeley, Ca. 94710

ZIEGLER, VICKIE, AND ELIZABETH CAMPBELL, eds. *Circle One: A Woman's Guide to Self-Health and Sexuality* (2nd ed., rev.), 1975.

> P.O. Box 7211
> Colorado Springs, Colo. 80933

HYSTERECTOMY AND MENOPAUSE

CHERRY, SHELDON H., M.D. *The Menopause Myth.* New York: Ballantine Books, 1976.
> *"A guide to understanding and enjoying feminine maturity."*[2] *Discusses fears and myths and presents menopause in light of medical, psychological and sociological truths.*

COHEN, MARCIA, "Needless Hysterectomies," *Ladies Home Journal,* 93:3 (March 1976), 88-91.

DEUTSCH, HELENE, *The Psychology of Women,* Vol. II. New York: Grune and Stratton, 1945.

GRAY, MADELINE, *The Changing Years.* New York: The New American Library, 1970.

> *Discussion of menstruation, menopause, hormones, physical and psychological changes. Good chapter entitled "Don't Rush Into Hysterectomy." Includes nutrition and exercises.*

---

[2]From the cover of Cherry's book.

HOLLENDER, M.H., "Hysterectomy and Feelings of Femininity," *Medical Aspects of Human Sexuality*, 3, 7, 1969.

NUGENT, NANCY, *Hysterectomy: A Complete Up-To-Date Guide to Everything About It and Why It May Be Needed.* Garden City, N.Y.: Doubleday and Co., Inc., 1976.

PAULSHOCK, BERNADINE Z., M.D., "What Every Woman Should Know About Hysterectomy," *Today's Health,* 54:2 (February 1976).

"A physician discusses the myths about and reasons for this most common of women's operations."

Public Affairs Pamphlets

22 East 38th Street
New York, N.Y. 10016

Titles such as "Understanding Your Menopause," "When You Grow Older," "Your Family's Health," "Middle Age—Threat or Promise."

RAPHAEL, BEVERLEY, "The Crisis of Hysterectomy," *Australian and New Zealand Journal of Psychiatry,* 6: 2 (June 1972), 106-15.

RODGERS, J., "Rush to Surgery: Hysterectomy," *N.Y. Times Magazine* (September 21, 1975), p. 34ff.

RODGERS, J. "Too Many Hysterectomies," *Time,* 93:39 (February 7, 1969).

WEIDEGER, PAULA, *Menstruation and Menopause.* New York: Alfred A. Knopf, 1976.

The subtitle, "The Physiology and Psychology, the Myth and the Reality," describes the contents of a book which says that the onset and loss of this bodily function should not deny a woman of a positive sense of personhood.

PHYSICAL AND EMOTIONAL HEALTH

AMERICAN CANCER SOCIETY *How to Examine Your Breasts; Facts about Cancer.*

BENSON, HERBERT, M.D., *The Relaxation Response.* New York: Avon Books, 1976.

"A simple meditative technique that has helped millions to cope with fatigue, anxiety and stress."

BOGERT, L.J., G.M. BRIGGS AND D.H. COLLOWAY, *Nutrition and Physical Fitness.* Philadelphia: W.B. Saunders Co., 1973.

DAVIS, M. EDWARD, *Menopause and Estrogens.* Chicago: Budlong Press Co., 1969.

> *Illustrated facial exercise program.*

Health Pamphlets
> Extension Service
> U.S. Dept. of Agriculture
> 14th Street and Independence Ave. S.W.
> Washington, D.C. 20250

KRANE, JESSICA, *How to Use Your Hands to Save Your Face.* New York: Cornerstone Library, 1976.

> *Facial massage and exercise programs and suggestions.*

MAYER, JEAN, *Health.* New York: D. Van Nostrand Co., 1974.

> *"No one can be counted as educated if he or she is ignorant of the basic facts of health . . . without sufficient knowledge a person cannot prevent disease or make full use of our system of medical care."[3] Chapters on the human body, sexuality, nutrition, preventive medicine, health and the community, delivery of health care.*

STARE, F.J. AND M. MCWILLIAMS, *Living Nutrition.* New York: John Wiley and Sons, 1973.

For additional books dealing with food and nutrition, write for list from:

> National Academy of Sciences
> Printing and Publishing Office
> 2101 Constitution Avenue
> Washington, D.C. 20418

SEXUALITY

BARBOUR, JAMES R., Academic Ed., *Focus: Human Sexuality.* Guilford, Conn.: Annual Editions, Dushkin Publishing Group, 1977.

> The Dushkin Publishing Group
> Sluice Dock, Guilford, Conn. 06437

COMFORT, ALEX, *The Joy of Sex.* New York: Simon and Schuster/Fireside, 1972.

---

[3]From the Preface of Mayer's book, p. v.

Also look for *reprints of articles on sexual biology; sexual behavior; sexual dilemmas; sexual development.*

MASTERS, WILLIAM H. AND VIRGINIA E. JOHNSON, *The Pleasure Bond.* Boston: Little, Brown and Co., 1974.

> *A new look at sexuality and commitment. How to keep alive the physical attraction that originally brought couples together. How sexual relationships can be strengthened and intensified as time goes by. The elements that enrich the act of sex and create the pleasure bond.*

Non-Sexism

GENERAL

BEM, SANDRA LIPSITZ, "Fluffy Women and Chesty Men," *Psychology Today,* 9: 4 (September 1975), 58-62.

> *"An experimenter in sex roles reports her work with the 35 percent of us who don't march to a sex-typed drummer."*

Psychology Today
Consumer Service Division
595 Broadway
New York, N.Y. 10012

CARMICHAEL, CARRIE, *Non-Sexist Childrearing.* Boston: Beacon Press, 1977.

> *". . . invaluable data from the experiences of families who are following deliberate strategies to free their children from the limitations of sexual stereotyping."*[4]

COHEN, MONROE, ed., *Childhood Education.* Association For Childhood Int'l.: 52: 4 (February, 1976).

> *Issue contains several excellent articles, and resources on the topic, "Overcoming Sex Role Stereotypes."*

---

[4]From *The Beacon,* supplement to *Unitarian Universalist World,* January 1977, p. 1.

EAGAN, ANDREA, *Why Am I So Miserable If These Are the Best Years of My Life?* Philadelphia: J.B. Lippincott Co., 1976.

> *A feminist teenage "advice" book for those who parent or otherwise work with adolescents.*

GOUGH, PAULINE B., "41 Ways to Teach About Sex Role Stereotyping," *Learning,* 5:5 January, 1977, 72-80.

> *A well-developed list of experiences for children which will help them examine their environment (including the media) critically. Includes an excellent resource list for materials.*

GRAMS, ARMIN, AND DEEDEE JAMESON, "Changing Roles for Women and Men," *Childhood Education,* 49: 4 (January, 1973), 184-90.

> *Examines influences which lock people into stereotypes and looks to today's need for flexible "human" roles.*

LARRICK, NANCY, AND EVE MERRIAM, *Male and Female Under 18.* New York: Avon Books, 1973.

> *Information which could be used for high school discussion groups.*

> The Feminist Book Mart
> 41-17 150th Street
> Flushing, New York 11355

MITCHELL, JOYCE S., *Free to Choose: Decision-Making for Young Men.* New York: Delacorte Press, 1976.

> *Companion volume to "Other Choices for Becoming a Woman," this book is written for boys and discusses a wide gamut of subjects, stressing education.*

MITCHELL, JOYCE S., *Other Choices for Becoming a Woman.* New York: Delacorte Press, 1974.

> *Written for junior high-age, discussing a wide gamut of subjects, including careers.*

> Know, Inc.
> P.O. Box 86031
> Pittsburgh, Pa. 15221

MOUSTAKAS, CLARK E., AND CERETA PERRY, *Learning to Be Free.* Englewood Cliffs, N.J.: Prentice-Hall, Inc., 1973.

> *An excellent book for developing self-awareness and techniques to help children be free. Contains lists of materials and resources, a bibliography of children's books, and a "selected professional bibliography".*

PECK, ELLEN, AND JUDITH SENDEROWITZ, *Pronatalism: The Myth of Mom and Apple Pie.* New York: Thomas Y. Crowell Co., 1974.

> *Some two dozen articles detail and document the influence of society's institutions on gender and sexuality.*

YOUNG CHILDREN

ANDREWS, JAN, *Fresh Fish and Chips.*
> *The mother goes fishing and catches different kinds of sea creatures.* From:

Canadian Women's Educational Press
280 Bloor St.
West Suite 305
Toronto, Ontario, Canada

FEMINISTS ON CHILDREN'S MEDIA, *Sexism in Children's Books: A Bibliography.*
> *Selected listing including textbooks and encyclopedias.*

Know, Inc.
P.O. Box 86031
Pittsburgh, Pa. 15221

JACOBS, CAROL, AND CYNTHIA EATON, "Sexism in the Elementary School," *Today's Education.* Washington, D.C.: *NEA Journal,* 61: 20-2 (December, 1972).

JAN, JUDY, BECKY, RIC, AND BOB, *Some Things You Just Can't Do by Yourself.*
> *A story of some of the ways people depend on each other.*

New Seed Press
P.O. Box 3016
Standford, Calif. 94305

KLAGSBRUN, FRANCINE, *Free To Be . . . You and Me.* New York: McGraw-Hill Book Co., 1974.

> *Conceived by Marlo Thomas; a collection of stories, songs, and poems for liberated children.*

Learn Me, Inc.
> 642 Grand Avenue
> St. Paul Minn.

> *A pre-kindergarten through high school catalog of over 700 items (books, records, puzzles, games, toys) is available from this store. Materials are evaluated in terms of sterotyped images.*

LOERCHER, DONNA, *Girls and Boys . . . Together.*

> *Comprehensive listing of non-fiction, fiction, and biographies from young child to young adult.*

> The Feminist Book Mart
> 162-11 Ninth Avenue
> Whitestone, N.Y. 11357

MONTGOMERY, CONSTANCE, *Vermont School Bus Ride.*

> Vermont Crossroads Press
> P.O. Box 333
> Waitsfield, Vt. 05673

PARRISH, BARB, *Families Grow in Different Ways.*

> *Story about having babies by adoption or pregnancy.*

> Before We Are Six
> 12 Bridgeport Road, East
> Waterloo, Ontario, Canada

Toy Review

> 383 Elliot Street
> Newton, Mass. 02164

Women's Action Alliance

> *This group has designed stereotype-free materials for early childhood.*

> Dept. "C"
> 370 Lexington Avenue
> New York, N.Y. 10017

Parenting

BRIGGS, DOROTHY CORKVILL, *Your Child's Self-Esteem.* New York: Doubleday and Co., Inc., Dolphin Books, 1975.

> *Provides parents with "a basic framework as a guide [to] help you live with your child so that he is emotionally healthy." Contains checklists and a bibliography.*

CHESS, STELLA, *Your Child Is a Person.* New York: Viking Press, 1972.

DREIKURS, RUDOLPH, AND VICKI SOLTZ, *Children: The Challenge.* New York: Hawthorn Books, 1976.

GORDON, THOMAS, *Parent Effectiveness Training.* New York: Plume (New American Library) 1975.

HARRIS, THOMAS A., M.D., *I'm Okay, You're Okay.* New York: Avon Books, 1967.

SATIR, VIRGINIA, *Peoplemaking.* Palo Alto, Ca.: Science and Behavior Books, Inc., 1972.

> *Helps with insights and suggestions for improving communicating in the family.*

WALTER, JAMES, ed. *The Family Coordinator. National Council on Family Relations,* 25: 4 (October, 1976).

> *"Special Issue: Fatherhood," contains twenty-one articles relating to fathering, includes a "Bibliography of Literature Related to Roles of Fathers."*

Consumerism

ANNAS, GEORGE J., *The Rights of Hospital Patients.* New York: Avon Books, 1975.

> *Handbook written in association with the American Civil Liberties Union. Covers informed consent, consultation, records, confidentiality.*

Consumer Reports: The Medicine Show. Mount Vernon, N.Y.: Consumers Union, 1970.

> *Articles on Plain Truths about Products for Common Ailments, Choosing a Family Doctor, Guides to a Good Hospital.*

CHISARI, FRANCIS, M.D., ROBERT NAKAMURA, M.D., AND LORENA THORUP, R.N. *The Consumers Guide to Health Care.* Boston: Little Brown and Co., 1976.

> *Discusses quality of medical care; how you can improve it; choosing a physician; choosing a hospital; lists services available (addresses included).*

Community Action Programs

> Office of Economic Opportunity
> 1200 Nineteenth St. N.W.
> Washington, D.C. 20036

> *"Community Action for Health Series" titles such as: Community Action; Consumer Action; Health Services Programs; Adult Education.*

Docubooks.

> *Special references on treatment, benefits, risks, and alternatives to procedures. Designed to help patient participate more actively in making decisions.* From:

> Health Communication, Inc.
> 52 W. Kellog Blvd.
> St. Paul, Minn 55102

Health Right.

> *A national women's health journal, issued quarterly; pamphlets also available.* From:

> Women's Health Forum
> 175 Fifth Avenue
> New York, New York 10010

How to Organize: "Woman's Right to Health."

> *A panel discussion kit developed by N.O.W.*

> The Baltimore Chapter
> National Organization of Women
> P.O. Box 21, Sunshine Avenue
> Keysville, Md. 21087

Indexes to health care and consumer pamphlets and list of GPO bookstores.

> Superintendent of Documents
> U.S. Government Printing Office
> Washington, D.C. 20402

> *See also Sylvia Porter, "Money Book," p. 1056.*

KENNEDY, EDWARD M. *In Critical Condition: The Crisis in America's Health Care.* New York: Simon and Schuster, 1972.

> *"Are you aware that millions of Americans who are sick or injured get no help at all? That the quality of health care varies widely. . . ? That Americans are paying today 170% more than in 1960?"⁵ Chapters on "What Price Good Health," The Medical Maze, The Health Insurance Trap, and Good Health Care: A Right for all Americans.*

Leadership Pamphlet Series

> Adult Education Association
> 1225 Nineteenth Street N.W.
> Washington D.C. 20036

> *Titles such as: Planning Better Programs; Guide to Planning Meetings; Talking Action in the Community.*

Medical Self-Care Magazine.

> Box 31549
> San Francisco, Ca. 94131

> *A self-help journal providing "access to medical tools," including consumer articles and health information. An excellent source. See especially issue no. 1, June 1976.*

---

⁵From the Introduction of Kennedy's book, p. 13.

Office For Community Health Centers

> Bureau of Community Health Services
> U.S. Public Health Service
> Department of Health, Education and Welfare
> 5600 Fishers Lane
> Rockville, Maryland 20852

NATIONAL COMMISSION ON COMMUNITY HEALTH SERVICES, *Health Is a Community Affair.* Cambridge, Mass.: Harvard University Press, 1966.

> *Report to the people of the United States "that the findings and recommendations considered here will give inspiration and guidance to communities everywhere." Chapters on health services, health manpower, the consumer, resources, and action planning.*

Organizing for Health Care: Source Catalog 3 by Source Collective.

> Beacon Press
> 25 Beacon Street
> Boston, Mass. 02106

PORTER, SYLVIA, *Money Book.* New York: Doubleday and Company, 1975.

> *Excellent chapters on shopping for health care, health insurance, rights as a consumer, where to get help. Section on resources with addresses.*

Prime Time

> *A monthly feminist publication for older women; includes articles on health.*

> 420 W. 46th St.
> New York, N.Y. 10036
> (212-265-5839)

SCIENTIFIC AMERICAN, *Life and Death and Medicine.* San Francisco: W.H. Freeman and Co., 1973.

> *Thirteen articles covering a wide range of contemporary health care issues ranging from "growing up" through chemical*

*intervention" to "The medical economy;" includes bib-
liographies.*

Shopper's Guide to Surgery

Consumer News Inc.
813 National Press Building
529 14th N.W.
Washington, D.C. 20045

Shopper's Guide to Health Insurance

Consumer News, Inc.
813 National Press Building
529 14th N.W.
Washington, D.C. 20045

Shopper's Guide to Surgery
Shopper's Guide to Dentistry
Shopper's Guide to Life Insurance, and others.

Pennsylvania State
Insurance Department
Harrisburg, Pa. 17120

Social Policy, "Special Health Issue."

*A bi-monthly magazine; proposes a consumer-intensive health
care model.*
Social Policy
184 Fifth Avenue
New York, N.Y. 10010

Source Book of Health Insurance and *Introduce Yourself to Health Insurance*

Health Insurance Institute
277 Park Avenue
New York, N.Y. 10017

See also: Porter, Sylvia, "Money Book," p. 236.

ROSENBERG, KEN, AND GORDON SCHIFF, eds., *The Politics of Health Care:
A Bibliography.*

An annotated sourcebook.
New England Free Press
60 Union Square
Somerville, Mass. 02143

TROELSTRUP, ARCH W., *The Consumer in American Society* (4th ed.). New York: McGraw-Hill Book Co., 1970.

> *An excellent book which covers a wide gamut of consumer information, includes a listing of Federal Consumer Agencies and Aids in Washington, D.C. Chapter 12, "Buying Good Health Care and Services," is highly recommended.*

Getting It Together

BEQUAERT, LUCIA, *Single Women: Alone and Together*. Boston: Beacon Press, 1976.

> *" . . . on the strategies millions of women have adopted to live free lives without marrying."*[6]

CLANTON, GORDON, AND LYNN G. SMITH, *Jealousy*. Englewood Cliffs, N.J.: Prentice-Hall, Inc., 1977.

COX, SUE, *Female Psychology: The Emerging Self*. Chicago: Science Research Associates, 1976.

> *Chapters on biological and psychological perspectives, feminism, sexuality, consciousness raising, what is a healthy woman? Lists of experiential exercises included.*

DAVITZ, JOEL AND LOIS DAVITZ, *Making It from Forty to Fifty*. New York: Random House, Inc., 1976.

GARDNER, JOHN, *Self-Renewal*. New York: Harper and Row, Publishers, 1964.

HAMMER, SIGNE, ed., *Women, Body and Culture*. New York: Harper and Row, Publishers (Perennial Library), 1975.

HARDING, M. ESTHER, *The Way of All Women*. New York: Harper Colophon Books, 1975.

> *Dr. C.G. Jung, who wrote the introduction, feels this book contributes to a "striving of our time for a deeper knowledge of the human being and for a clarification of the confusion existing in the relationship between the sexes."*

---

[6]From *The Beacon,* supplement to *Unitarian Universalist World,* January 1977, p. 1.

JONGEWARD, DOROTHY, *Women as Winners.* Reading, Mass.: Addison-Wesley Pub. Co., Inc., 1976.

> *"A tool for women who are about to decide to be productive, to be important, to learn new and interesting skills." Chapters include: Steps to Awareness; Appreciating Your Body and Your Femininity; Daring to Dream; Contracting for Personal Growth.*

KOHL, HERBERT, *Half the House.* New York: Bantam Books, Inc., 1976.

> *The author of "36 Children" and "Reading, How To" shares his personal growth experiences around the question, "Is it possible to change oneself in midlife despite the practical pressures to survive?"*

HOWELL, MARY C., *Helping Ourselves: Families and the Human Network.* Boston: Beacon Press, 1975.

> *An inspiring message from a pediatrician and mother, helping us to develop faith in our potential to assume responsibilities for ourselves.*

LOPATA, HELENA Z., *Occupation: Housewife.* London: Oxford University Press, 1971.

OTTO, HERBERT A. AND JOHN MANN, eds., *Ways of Growth.* New York: Pocket Books, 1971.

> *A collection of articles, suggested by Abraham Maslow, by pioneering professionals in the human potential movement.*

RAMEY, JAMES, *Intimate Friendships.* Englewood Cliffs, N.J.: Prentice-Hall, Inc., 1976.

> *Examines the ways we do or do not develop the ability to form close non-possessive alliances with others. Good for the adult who wishes to become more free.*

RODGERS, CARL, *On Becoming a Person.* Boston: Houghton Mifflin Co., 1965.

RONCO, WILLIAM, *Jobs: How People Create Their Own.* Boston: Beacon Press, 1977.

> *" . . . describes how many people today are managing to do just what they want to do with their lives, and get paid for it."*

SEYMOUR, JOHN, *The Guide to Self-Sufficiency.* London: The Hearst Corp. and Dorling Kindsersley Ltd., 1976.

Specific information and resources to help you develop greater competency in many aspects of your daily life.

SHEEHY, GAIL, *Passages: Predictable Crises of Adult Life.* New York: E.P. Dutton and Co., 1976.

Chapters on the Life Cycle, Pulling Up Roots, and on passage from the twenties, to the thirties, forties, and on to renewal.

SINACORE, JOHN S., AND ANGELA C. SINACORE, *Introductory Health: A Vital Issue.* New York: Macmillan Pub. Co. Inc., 1975.

"There is a growing realization that the kind of lifestyle a person leads may promote health—the decisions a person makes as to how he will live can be more important than any actions a doctor may try . . ." Chapters on maintaining personal health; human relationships and family life; health and the consumer.

TAUBMAN, BRYNA, *How to Become an Assertive Woman.* New York: Pocket Books, 1976.

How your body and actions convey your image; how to assess potential; how to handle problems; how to take action.

VIORST, JUDITH, *How Did I Get to Be 40 and Other Atrocities.* New York: Simon and Schuster, 1976.

VIORST, JUDITH, *It's Hard to Be Hip Over Thirty and Other Tragedies of Married Life.* New York: Simon and Schuster, 1968.

AUDIO-VISUAL MATERIALS

The film prices given here are correct as of this writing.

How About You?

Texture Films
1600 Broadway

Room 604A
New York, N.Y. 10023

Shows a discussion of feelings about sexuality, including birth control information, in a high school setting. (Rental: $35.00.)

How To Make a Woman.

Polymorph Films
331 Newbury St.
Boston, Ma. 02115

A powerful adaptation of an award-winning play illuminating the mechanism of personal and sexual relationships between men and women. It is not an objective balancing of arguments but a passionate, dramatic statement about women's subjugation and a unique, effective plea for understanding. Suitable for college and adult audiences with discussion after viewing. (58 mins., color; rental: $60.00; purchase: $595.00.)

Sex Education Films.

Multi-Media Resource Center
330 Ellis
San Francisco, Ca. 94108

A series of several sex education films. Information is available at the above address.

Self-Health.

Multi-Media Resource Center
540 Powell St.
San Francisco, Ca. 94108

Shows women sharing education about self-examination. (Rental: $40.00; $20.00 for women's groups.)

Taking Our Bodies Back: The Women's Health Movement.

Cambridge Documentary Films, Inc.
P.O. Box 385
Cambridge, Ma. 02139

Gives information about many women's health care issues as well as showing how many women are now a part of the health care movement. (Rental: $39.00.)

Why Jane Can't Win.

> Oregon Education Association
> 6900 S.W. Haines Rd.
> Tegard, Ore. 97223
>
> *Current textbooks are examined in terms of sex role stereotyping and suggestions for action are given in this slide/tape film. (Rental: $17; $35 for 5 days.)*

Anything They Want to Be.

> *Shows the crippling effect of sex role stereotyping in kindergarten on the eventual limitations on competency and career development of females. (Rental: $12.00; 7 minutes.)*

"Free To Be . . . You and Me," sponsored by Ms. Foundation.

> *A record album presenting 22 selections by celebrities (such as Marlo Thomas, Carl Reiner, Carol Channing, Roosevelt Grier, Diana Ross), singing songs for liberated young people.*

Hey! What About Us?

> *Gives insight into sex role stereotyping in physical activities in elementary schools. (Rental: $17.00; 15 minutes.)*

I Is For Important.

> *Shows negative effects of sex role stereotyping in social interactions on children grades K-8. (Rental: $15.00; 12 minutes.)*

In All Fairness.

> University of California
> Extension Media Center
> Berkeley, Ca. 94720
>
> *A handbook which presents study guides to the preceding three films (above) and a bibliography is included. Extra copies may be purchased.*

A Better Place To Stand.

> *Shows how people can live successfully with one another and stabilize healthy and happy relationships. (Virginia Satir). ($50 preview rental; 19 minutes.)*

Insights.

    Manitou Programs, Inc.
    4900 IDS Center
    Minneapolis, Mn. 55402

    Dramatizes the vital subject of self-worth. Four different characters describe how they developed a strong sense of self-worth. Film includes "The Ballad of Gerald" which underlines the importance of a sense of self-worth to a child and an entire family. ($50 preview rental; 19 minutes.)

Sugar and Spice.

    Odeon Films
    22 West 48th Street
    New York, N.Y. 10026

    Show what parents and teachers are doing to eliminate sex role stereotypes both in the home and in day care centers and schools. (Rental: $10; 32 minutes.)

Unlearning Sex Roles.

    Resource Options
    1916 Napa Avenue
    Berkeley, Ca. 94707
    415-527-8483

    Helps to illustrate the degree of sex role socialization that children bring to the classroom, to expand possible role options, and to extend the skills which children of either sex need in order to assume expanded social roles. (30 minute video tape in b/w; ½" portapak; ¾" cassette; rental: $35.)

Women's Rights in the U.S.

    Altana Films
    340 East 34th Street
    New York, N.Y. 10016

    The myth of female inferiority is deeply ingrained in society. This film documents the growth of women's opposition to this myth and links the past with the current feminist movement. (Rental: $40; 27 minutes.)

Self-Help Gynecological Slide Show.
  Available from Feminist Women's Health Centers at

746 South Crenshaw 429 South Sycamore St.
Los Angeles, Ca. 90005 Santa Ana, Ca. 92701
(213-936-7219) (714-547-0327)

444 48th Street
Oakland, Ca. 94706
(415-653-2130)

PAKS (Program Awareness Kits).

Mr. Edward J. Palmer
Action for Independent Maturity (AIM)
1909 K Street, N.W.
Washington, D.C. 20049
(202-872-4943)

*"Short form, multi-media presentations on subjects of high
'middle years' interest." Includes film, guidebook of resources
and exercises, and a program leader's manual.*

Back to School, Back to Work.

American Personnel and Guidance Assn.
Film Department
1607 New Hampshire Ave. N.W.
Washington, D.C. 20009
(202-483-4633)

*A film by Joan Pearlman which can help women and their
family members as the woman assumes an additional role.
(#77540, 20 minutes; 16mm. in color; rental: $25 a day, $250
purchase. 24-page leader's guide available for $2.75, #72051.)
An excellent film—recipient of the 1975 National Council on
Family Relations Family Life Film Award.*

Men in Nurturing Roles.

N.A.E.Y.C.
1834 Connecticut Ave.
Washington, D.C. 20009

*A set of four poster-size photographs of men in nurturing
roles.*

Patient's Bill of Rights[1]

You have the right:

1. To considerate and respectful care.

2. To get complete information from your physician concerning your diagnosis, treatment and prognosis in terms you understand.

3. To receive whatever information you think is necessary to give your informed advance consent for any procedure and/or treatment.

4. To every consideration for your privacy concerning your medical care program.

---

[1]From The American Hospital Association.

5. To refuse treatment to the extent permitted by law, and to be informed of the medical consequences of your action. This means you have a right to die if your condition is hopeless.

6. To expect that all communications and records pertaining to your care will be treated as confidential.

7. To expect a hospital to respond, within reason, to your request for services.

8. To get information about any relationship between your hospital and other health care and educational institutions in so far as your care is concerned; and to get information (including names) on the existence of any professional relationship between individuals who are treating you.

9. To be advised if the hospital proposes to engage in or perform human experimentation on you in the course of your care or treatment.

10. To expect reasonable continuity of care.

11. To examine and receive an explanation of your bill, regardless of the source of payment.

12. To know what hospital rules and regulations apply to your conduct as a patient.

Glossary

ADHESIONS. Fibrous or scar tissue that may form following infection or surgery and which unites two surfaces that are normally separated.

ADRENAL GLAND. An endrocrine gland which lies on top of each kidney.

ANEMIA. A deficiency in the blood, usually of red blood cells, which deprives tissues of adequate oxygen.

BIOPSY. Removal and examination of tissue from anywhere in the body. Usually done as a diagnostic aid to determine the cause of a growth or a tumor.

CARDIOVASCULAR. Pertaining to the heart and blood vessels.

CATHETER. Any rubber, plastic, or metal tube used to drain or to instill fluids through a body passage.

CERVIX.   The lower neck-like portion of the uterus which opens into the vagina and serves as a passageway between the two organs.

CURETTAGE.   The cleansing of a diseased surface with a small surgical instrument called a curette.

CYSTOCELE.   Prolapse of the urinary bladder into the vagina.

D & C.   Dilatation and Curettage. Enlarging the opening in the cervix with a dilatating instrument in order to permit scraping the walls of the uterus, to cleanse the surface or obtain tissue for study.

DOUBLE STANDARD.   The moral code which allows greater sexual permissiveness and gratification for males than females.

ENDOCRINE.   Refers to glands that regulate body activity by secreting hormones into the blood.

ENDOMETRIOSIS.   A condition in which tissue normally found lining the uterus is found growing on other pelvic organs or locations in the pelvic cavity.

ENDOMETRIUM.   The membrane lining of the uterus.

FIBROID TUMORS.   Common benign tumors of the uterus named for tissue which resembles fibers. Also called myoma.

HIDDEN AGENDAS. The real goals which are camouflaged by what is overtly stated. Example: "What color are your sneakers?" is really intended either to find out if the child knows her colors, or to make her feel "smart." Hopefully, it is not intended to gain information as it is assumed that the adult knows his or her colors.

HORMONE. A secretion from a gland, organ, or tissue which, when released into the bloodstream, acts as a chemical messenger to body organs to stimulate or retard a life process. Examples: insulin, thyroid, estrogen.

INTRAVENOUS (IV). The administration of fluids through a vein.

MENARCHE. The establishment or beginning of menstrual functioning (menstruation.)

MENOPAUSE. The period of time during which the menstrual cycle decreases and stops and the ovaries gradually cease functioning.

OSTEOPOROSIS. Thinning or inadequate absorption of calcium into the bone.

OVULATION. The process by which an egg is discharged from the ovary into the fallopian tube, usually occurring midway between menstrual periods.

PATHOLOGY. The scientific study of anatomic or functional changes caused (produced) by disease.

PESSARY. A device placed in the vagina to support the uterus.

PITUITARY GLAND. The master gland of the endocrine system which controls hormone production. It lies at the base of the brain.

PROLAPSE.   The falling down—or downward displacement—of an organ.

RECTOCELE.   Protrusion of part of the rectum into the vagina.

SELF-ACTUALIZING.   In Abraham Maslow's "hierarchy of needs" theory, the self-actualizing person is one who is able to develop what has been achieved, once other needs have been met (physical, safety, belonging, and esteem.) The self-actualizer is not motivated in the ordinary sense of the word. Rather, he or she takes the initiative to implement the fulfillment of his or her potential.

SEXUALITY.   The total of one's sexual self as it relates to sensual and sexual activity, gender identity, and role adoption.

VASOMOTOR.   Effecting a change on the consistency of blood vessels.

Index